MAKING MIRACLES

MAKING MIRACLES

AN
EXPLORATION
INTO THE
DYNAMICS OF
SELF-HEALING

Dr. Paul C. Roud

Introduction by Bernie Siegel

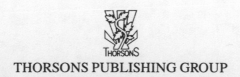

THORSONS PUBLISHING GROUP

In a few cases identifying information, including names
of persons and places, has been disguised
to honor the individual's request for anonymity.

This UK edition first published 1990
First published in the United States by
Warner Books, Inc., 666 Fifth Avenue, New York, NY 10103

British Library Cataloguing in Publication Data

Roud, Paul C.
    Making miracles: an exploration
    into the dynamics of self-healing.
    1. Mental healing
    I. Title
    615.851

ISBN 0-7225-2427-7

*Published by Thorsons Publishers Limited,
Wellingborough, Northamptonshire NN8 2RQ, England.*

Printed and Bound in Great Britain by
Hartnolls Limited, Bodmin, Cornwall.

10 9 8 7 6 5 4 3 2 1

To my mother, Bernice Roud,
the first person to teach me about courage and love

ACKNOWLEDGMENTS

Ellen Grobman's intelligence, sensitivity, and love made this project possible.

Professor Jack Wideman's faith that I would find my own way was the original source of this work. The message from professors Ted Slovin and Don Banks—that the pursuit of academic excellence could happily coexist with the spiritual quest—brought meaning and joy to my journey.

Some kind and very caring physicians provided instrumental technical support: Paul Flandreau, Sid Baker, Dave Sherman, Bernie Siegel, Paul Berman, Wayne Gavryck, Steve Eipper, and Kit French.

I am grateful to friends Michael Shandler, Gail Shufrin, Steve Berman, Barbara Levy, Eva Gumprecht, Nina Shandler, Steve Orlov, Sebern Fisher, Margaret Gosselin, Debbie Abrams, and others. For years, they listened to my thoughts and questions about extraordinary survivors. Their conviction that the work was valuable sustained me and the project during some very difficult moments.

The book wouldn't have been written without Agnes Birnbaum's dogged perseverance. It wouldn't have been as good or as accessible without Fredda Isaacson's editorial guidance.

Thanking the survivors is a bit overwhelming. In many ways, my role (when done well) was merely to function as the intermediary who would make their accounts available to others. The survivors shared a vision of the possibilities that exist for all of us. By offering this glimpse, my life has been profoundly changed.

CONTENTS

I do not believe healing is a coincidence. I have found that the patient who makes what is considered to be a miraculous recovery has almost always made some drastic change toward a more loving and accepting life-style.

Miracles happen at the unconscious, archetypal level; they don't come from the cold intellect. That is one reason why doctors have trouble "seeing" miracles. To see, you have to be able to believe. In medical school, you're taught to treat everyone as a statistic. If something occurs that doesn't fit the statistical profile, you do not "see" it. In cases where the patient has done amazingly well, nobody gives the patient credit and says the patient has accomplished something unique. Instead, doctors wonder if this was an error in diagnosis. When the case can't be dismissed as a misdiagnosis, the exceptional recovery is labeled a "spontaneous remission," a phrase that teaches doctors nothing about the recovery and stimulates no inquiry into the causes behind it. A Mount Everest of knowledge goes unexplored because the medical establishment says it's not there. Success has never been studied.

In writing and talking about exceptional patients, I have had the opportunity to meet many people who were cured of supposedly incurable diseases. I consider the exploration of these people and their

MAKING MIRACLES

experiences important work that can benefit us all. There is a vital need to knock on the doors of the people who have pulled themselves back from the edge of death and ask, "What did you do? How did you feel? Why do you think you did so well? Why didn't you die when you were supposed to?"

That is the beauty of *Making Miracles*; Paul Roud listened carefully while survivors told him their stories. The essence of the survivors' experiences is related in their own words, and an insightful and evocative interpretation of their experience follows. I support his request that you not stop there but integrate their stories and figure out what meaning they have for you, for there is always a lesson behind the story of those who do incredibly well. It is no accident, no lucky break, no "spontaneous remission." They tell us they worked damn hard at not dying. They made choices, they changed their lives psychologically and spiritually, and they learned how to face fear. They find a reason to go on; they want to continue to love and create meaning in their lives.

I want to remind people that there's a 100 percent mortality associated with life. Some people give themselves an incredible burden, thinking, "If I work hard enough in therapy, love myself enough, or meditate enough, then I'll be sure to live forever." That is an absurdity and sets one up for failure. You can't cure everything. There's so much we don't understand about the unconscious and its relationship to healing. You can love, jog, and eat vegetables—and still die. The message is: Heal your life and the by-product will be physical. The question is not "Why me?"; instead the attitude should be "Try me."

Paul Roud's interviews bear out what I have observed in my own practice. The fundamental problem most patients face, that all of us face, is an inability to love ourselves because we have been unloved by others during some crucial part of our lives. If somebody else loves us unconditionally, it may help us realize that we are lovable. Therefore a fundamental element of my relationship with my patients is to love them unconditionally, because I know that, if I can do this, they may discover their own self-worth, their own self-love. Positive emotions change your body's biochemistry, and that can lead to physical healing as a by-product.

To a surgeon, suffering is no abstraction. It's right there in front of you in the hospital room or on the operating table. If one sees, one can witness how nobly and beautifully people are going through their pain. Their handicaps and disabilities are exposed: They may be missing parts of their bodies, tubes everywhere, and yet, when you look in their eyes, they're still glowing and alive. One sees their wholeness, not their disability, and they are "strong at the broken places." They are healed, if not cured. It's possible to fall in love with individuals in a minute because they're so inspiring. I believe that this is the essence of the healing relationship between doctor and patient. As I learned from *The Velveteen Rabbit*, once you are real you can't be ugly except to those who don't understand.

One of the most important contributions of this book is that it verifies what our hearts already know—there is always reason for hope. Faith is healing, and the people of *Making Miracles* demonstrate how powerful it can be. They believe in possibilities, not probabilities. It's important to believe in your treatment and then to proceed with a positive attitude. Conflict is what wears you out. When you choose your form of healing, when you're at peace with your physician and your treatment, your body responds very differently than if you're in conflict. When patients have faith in me and see the relationship as a healing experience, they come through their operation without pain. Their faith heals them, and then I get credit for being a wonderful surgeon.

You may read *Making Miracles* to find answers for yourself or to help someone else. Either way, I think you will discover a fundamental truth that applies to both the sick and the well. Love makes life worth living, no matter how long it lasts. I feel it also increases the likelihood of physical healing, but that is a bonus. The idea is to love because it feels good, not because it will help us live forever. But please don't wait for a catastrophe to awaken you.

The problem isn't that we don't know the path; the problem is how to get on it. Spirituality, unconditional love, and the ability to see that pain and problems are opportunities for growth and redirection—these things allow us to make the best of the time we have. Then we realize the present moment is all we have, but it is infinite.

There's an old Indian saying: "When you were born, you cried and the whole world rejoiced. Live such a life that when you die, the whole world cries and you rejoice."

BERNIE S. SIEGEL, M.D.

I did not arrive at my understanding of the fundamental laws of the Universe through my rational mind.

Albert Einstein

INTRODUCTION

Five years ago, doctors told my father that his prostate cancer, a disease that had been controlled for nearly a decade, was spreading. The cancer had metastasized to his kidney, liver, and, most horribly, his skull. The doctors explained that there was nothing more that they could do—he would die shortly. Certainly the physicians agreed, there was nothing the patient or family could do. The task, it seemed, was to help him die comfortably.

My family conferred uneasily, questioning whether we should encourage my father to see a different specialist or try an "alternative" approach. We wondered about nutritional programs, acupuncture, and imaging. But, far more seasoned in matters of terminal illness, the experts did not waver. There was no hope, they said. So mostly we just waited.

After my father's death, a nagging question lingered in my mind: Does anyone survive a "terminal" illness?

The answer I found is yes. A small number of terminal patients do survive; a few even go on to lead normal lives. In fact, there are rare patients who actually become totally free of disease. The people in this book are living proof.

To some, these documented cases appear miraculous. For the more scientifically oriented, they represent "a significant aberration from medically established norms." These differing points of view, though, are unimportant compared to the consensus most will share after reading these accounts. Mere chance or good fortune does not appear to be the reason for such sensational medical recoveries. It seems the patients made their miracles happen.

Before attempting to accomplish anything great, it is customary first to learn from people who have successfully walked the path before. After their teachings have been integrated in a personally meaningful way, we then put heart and soul into achieving the desired goal.

Yet to recover from serious illness we generally act as though, except for going to the doctor, it is best to remain passive while waiting to see what will happen. Even after someone is told that Western medicine can do no more, rarely will a person seek out others who have recovered from the same disease. There is, of course, no guarantee that extraordinary survivors will offer anything of value. But given how little there is to lose, why haven't we attempted to learn from them?

Part of the explanation is simple. Many people don't realize that extraordinary recoveries really do happen. The primary purpose of *Making Miracles* is to bridge this information gap. The following pages tell the stories of men and women who have conquered overwhelming medical odds. Many were diagnosed with terminal cancer and given less than a couple of years to live. One woman's lung cancer had metastasized, making it practically impossible for her to breathe. The family was warned to prepare for her imminent death. Today this woman leads a normal life as a homemaker and mother. One man regained the use of his legs after spending twenty years paralyzed in a wheelchair.

Norman Cousins, celebrated for his personal cure from a degenerative connective tissue disease (which he wrote about in *Anatomy of an Illness*), discusses his recovery from an illness even more lethal. Cousins's family doctor wrote, "I confess that I myself find it difficult to believe that anyone who has been hit by a myocardial infarction and congestive heart failure could have come through the experience as he has done." All of the people included in this book have done much better than authoritative medical opinion predicted, though not all of the medical battles have been resolved. Two people discuss their remarkable ongoing struggles.

A woman's total recovery from severe mental illness gives tender witness to the healing power of love and hope. Despite suicide attempts that were narrowly averted, a life-threatening loss of weight from anorexia nervosa, and a very poor prognosis, this woman is now bedrock sane.

Medical science grossly understates the incidence of extraordinary recovery. For example, medical texts aver that spontaneous regression of cancer is exceedingly rare, occurring only once every 60,000 to 100,000 cases. (Regression is considered spontaneous when a malignant tumor disappears or shrinks significantly and medical treatment cannot adequately account for the improved condition.) However, the number of individuals I was able to locate with medically unexplainable cancer regression indicates that the phenomenon is significantly more common than supposed. Researchers from the Netherlands, Marc J. de Vries, M.D., Ph.D., and Daan C. van Baalen, M.D., corroborate these impressions. Based on research just released, these medical faculty members believe that spontaneous regression is much more frequent than the literature asserts because of the "relative ease" with which they found seven cases for their own study. Most exceptional histories fail to reach public notice because, unlike these cases, they are never recorded in medical journals or anyplace else.

Another factor keeps the count down. If a person is diagnosed with a serious illness and then the illness disappears without medical intervention considered sufficient to eliminate the illness, professionals often conclude that the individual must have been misdiagnosed.

Since medical science knows that some extraordinary patients exist, whatever the exact number, why hasn't there been an attempt to learn from this population? Every year the United States government alone spends more than $2 billion on cancer research, more than $500 million on heart disease research, and more than $250 million on mental illness research, with relatively little success. Yet a small group of people exist who did much better than experts ever anticipated, and no one thinks to ask them how they did it.

Because medical thinking today views the mind and body as separate and distinct entities, it is easy to see how such a monumental oversight continues. According to this conventional view, the conscious mind can not significantly influence physical well-being. A patient therefore must be powerless to deliberately affect his or her healing. Thoughts, feelings, and behavior that stem from a patient's intuitive sense of what will heal his or her body are considered irrelevant to the disease process. The successes of the extraordinary patient are seen as statistical quirks, random events beyond any individual's control. Consequently, there is no reason to think that these people have anything of value to teach researchers, doctors, or other patients. They have simply been lucky.

Norman Mages, a professor of psychology, and Gerald Mendelsohn, a professor of psychiatry, speaking to a professional audience about cancer, describe the prevalent attitude toward serious illness in general:

> Though located in one's body, cancer is in a psychological sense external to the self. It cannot be understood (or affected) by introspection; rather it is through medical diagnostic procedures and the technical knowledge of others that a patient obtains information about the nature, seriousness, and likely progression of the problems to be faced. Furthermore, since the physical changes produced by cancer are not a product of one's thoughts or feelings, they cannot be made to go away nor can they be controlled by internal mental operations such as repression or sublimation. This does not mean that patients must remain completely passive, but it does mean that they must act through others, namely the appropriate medical personnel.

Such assertions, which reflect conventional medical thought, are remarkable statements for people of science whose expertise is the mind, for no one has gathered significant data to show that thoughts and feelings are unrelated to cancer development and its progression. In fact, there is little evidence and absolutely no proof that emotions are unrelated to most major illnesses.

Professionals who dogmatically insist that psychological factors have no impact on serious illness, with nothing to back up the claim except historical precedent, indicate how threatening this arena is to the medical establishment. The possibility that some patients themselves engineered their extraordinary recoveries represents the quintessential threat. A survivor of acute monocytic and myelocytic leukemia personally knows how disorienting an experience such as hers can be to a medical scientist. She explained: "My father's a scientist. He can't deal with my recovery. It's right there in the biology textbooks, in the technical papers: Nobody lives through the experiences I had. He loves me very much. I'm his daughter. But my recovery just pulls the pins right out from under all of his research."

Many of the extraordinary survivors are incredulous that they have not become the focus of medical curiosity. Oftentimes their doctors, the same ones who had previously told them that they would die in the near future, did not even ask their special patients a single question about what had happened to them. A woman whose survival was classified by an oncologist as a 1-in-1,000 possibility described her doctor's response to the course of her illness:

> He seemed wary of me even though the cancer was not growing nearly as fast as he thought it would. But rather than being delighted for me, he seemed upset by it.
>
> It was very disturbing for me to go to see the doctors. I wanted to talk with somebody who was in a powerful position in regard to my health, who was invested in whatever might work. I wanted to share with them the things that I was doing. Instead, I felt like I was fighting the authorities. I never felt they were really on my side or that they wanted to work with me. I think that's when I decided that I needed alternatives.

After trying a host of alternative approaches, she decided it would be best to find an oncologist to follow her case. Her experience with the new doctor, however, was not very different from the last one:

> When I first started seeing this latest oncologist, he was very belligerent. He thought I was a crazy woman.
>
> He constantly tells me that somehow I am different. My cancer is not responding like anybody else's he has seen. It's a very slow-growing kind of cancer—so far. He makes sure to tell me this all the time. I don't appreciate it.
>
> He says, "You've got to take this. There's nothing else that works, you're just into denial." I feel like he's angry with me. He frightens me quite a bit. Every time I go there, he says, "Are you ready to take the Tamoxifen now?" And I say, "No."
>
> I know that when I leave there, he's not feeling that great. He wants to give me something. When he can't give me something, I think it makes him feel helpless. I feel like I'm doing something bad to him. It's an awful feeling.
>
> Every once in a while I say to myself, "I'm never going

back to see him.'' But then I laugh and say, ''Well, maybe this man will finally learn something from this.''

When this woman attempted to confront her physician about the way she was feeling, he immediately referred her to a different doctor. The threat that keeps a physician from delighting in a patient's unexpected success, like the threat that prevents a father/scientist from unambivalently rejoicing over his daughter's return to health, runs deep.

A brief historical overview helps explain how the idea that the body and mind are separate entities developed into such a powerful medical model. Eventually this model may seem no closer to the truth than the ancient belief that illness was the result of spirit intervention. But the idea did take hold for good reason. It was a way of seeing nature that paved the path for spectacular medical successes.

Our ancestors had an appreciation, however primitive, of the holistic nature of disease. Healers relied on the total environment, especially the patient's beliefs, attitudes, and personal relationships, to promote health. But beginning around the sixteenth century, medical explorers began to learn more about the autonomous functioning of the circulatory, respiratory, and digestive systems. Regardless of the technical accuracy of their ''discoveries,'' the effort to determine how specific components of the body work meant that the body could no longer be considered an indivisible whole. In the seventeenth century, René Descartes said that the best way to understand a disease was to study its most basic form, removed from other influences. The belief that disease was a localized malfunction, a breakdown of a specific part of the body, flourished with the advent of surgery. Beginning around 1850, the use of anesthetics made it increasingly common for physicians to remove or fix whatever body piece was not working properly.

Less than forty years later, it was discovered that certain infectious diseases were transmitted through microorganisms. Steven Locke, M.D., and Douglas Colligan explain what happened from there:

Diseases that had been the scourge of humankind were dropping before one magic bullet after another. In 1911 researchers developed a special arsenic compound, Salvarson, that effectively treated many forms of syphilis. In the 1920s insulin was isolated and insulin injections were extending the lifetime of diabetic patients. In the 1930s sulfa drugs appeared and, with them, cures for bacterial pneumonia, meningitis, gonorrhea, and urinary tract infections. By the 1940s the sulfa drugs were largely replaced by even more potent drugs, the antibiotics, made possible by the discovery of penicillin. It seemed that there was no disease that medical science could not handle.

The promise was not just a cure for all that ails us. The lure for consumers was cure without any need for their involvement or psychic sweat. All they had to do was take a pill or submit to an operation. Our sense of responsibility and personal power were surrendered willingly in return for a guarantee of health.

But the promise could not be kept. Medical science has had little success in eliminating or even controlling illnesses that are the major causes of death and disability today. Cancer, heart disease, arthritis, alcoholism, mental illness, and chronic respiratory illnesses rage on with little hope of significant progress in the near future.

Because conventional medical thinking has failed to explain, let alone cure, our modern plagues, it faces growing disenchantment. A new medical model, one that respects the whole person, is necessary to address our greatest medical challenges. The major illnesses are not going to be conquered without incorporating the psychological and spiritual dimensions of human life, along with the physical ones. Factors such as life-style, nutrition, relationships, and even our capacity to love and be loved must be explored before we will realize another new dawn in healing.

Conventional medical thinking, however, is making neither a quick nor graceful exit. Nor should we expect it to, for the past achievements of medical science have been great, and those who have accrued power and prestige from these past successes are invested in maintaining the status quo. Physicians who can expertly ply their science to help heal the sick may lack the human skills necessary to mobilize psychological and spiritual factors that heal. In order to potentiate these intangible but real healing factors, the doctor must be involved in a meaningful and caring relationship with the patient.

Unfortunately applicants are not accepted into medical schools on the basis of their psychological maturity or compassion, or because they are spiritually evolved human beings. Medical students aren't trained in the art of communications that heal or supervised about the best way to nurture the "inner wisdom" of their patients. The vast majority of physicians have a wide pool of scientific knowledge to draw from; most can competently analyze and synthesize the objective physiological facts. But extraordinary healing calls on factors beyond the rational mind.

Large and powerful institutions such as medical schools, drug companies, governmental agencies, and hospitals also have a major stake in keeping the health care system basically unchanged. Conducting research or practicing medicine in a manner heretical to certain entrenched principles, such as the mind/body split, incurs professional risk. As a result of these pressures, some professionals believe that psychological efforts to influence recovery must proceed covertly.

Charles Weinstock, M.D., conducted one of the rare research projects on spontaneous regression of cancer. He concluded that psychiatric therapies could "vastly improve the duration of life," but he candidly acknowledged, "The psychiatrist is warned, however, that he will meet much prejudice from the medical profession and would do best to emphasize the palliative [pain-relieving] nature of his interest and not to mention to the physician the hopes for deeper changes."

Weinstock published his work in a credible but esoteric medical journal. Editorial control of the major medical journals is the vehicle used by conventional medicine to guarantee that only ideas consistent with present ideology will be widely disseminated. Ultimately a major journal's authority to accept or reject research is the way that conventional medicine sanctifies some research as medical fact and relegates other ideas to the status of folklore.

Consider how the *New England Journal of Medicine* (NEJM), arguably the most prestigious medical journal in the world, has covered—or, more accurately, not covered—the topic of extraordinary survival. In June 1985, the national press, as it often does, reported on research that appeared in the NEJM. Many of the country's major newspapers ran such headlines as "Study Says Psychological Factors Have No Impact on Cancer." The researchers of this study, after investigating 359 patients with advanced cancer, concluded: "The inherent biology of the disease alone determines the prognosis, overriding the potentially mitigating influence of psychosocial factors." In other words, once a person has contracted advanced cancer, he or she is helpless to alter the course of the illness.

If you had cancer at the time, you probably remember the study. In my own psychotherapy with cancer patients, the news report of the research was devastating for a couple of people. Science had "proven" that they were powerless to influence the disease. The research "finding" led these people to feel helpless and profoundly depressed.

The sanctity of the NEJM is such that questioning of its research reports is seldom undertaken. In fact, however, one need not dig too deeply to realize that the findings in this instance cannot be substantiated.

The researchers administered psychological interviews to people shortly after they were diagnosed with advanced cancer. They then investigated whether there was any correlation between patient longevity (or time until relapse) and how these subjects responded to the questionnaires. Since no correlation was found, the researchers concluded that psychological and social factors had no influence on the illness.

To understand the experiment, imagine that you have just been informed that you have advanced cancer, and the disease is expected to kill you relatively soon. While still reeling from the news, researchers ask you to complete some questionnaires. They ask about your satisfaction with your job, the quality of your social relationships, and how hopeless and helpless you feel, as well as about your satisfaction with life in general. The researchers assume that they have captured a psychological profile of who you are through these questions, even though, within the past three weeks, you have been given the most devastating news of your life. Most important, they don't allow for the possibility that your feelings may change in the coming months. Soon you may gather your personal resources, rediscover the beauty in your life, appreciate your strengths, and find reason to stay alive. But the researchers have no way of knowing this. They never interview you or anyone else again. Based on their initial interview, they conclude that attitudes don't affect illness.

You need not be a psychologist or psychiatrist to realize that your emotions are likely to fluctuate wildly in the weeks that follow the discovery of a lethal illness. Apparently the researchers and the editors of the NEJM never considered that the results of psychological interviews conducted with individuals who have just been given a terminal prognosis reflect a psychologically unique, volatile time in a person's life that is subject to dramatic change in the near future. The research design was based on the premise that humans are basically static, unchanging organisms.

In the following stories, survivors discuss the evolution of their psychological states. At first, most were in great distress after learning the prognosis. But this initial response was different from their emotional status a few months later. When these individuals were confronted with life-threatening illnesses, the most profound psychological change became possible. A man in his seventies who struggled successfully with lung cancer explained, "At first, I felt that if my time had come, it would behoove me to recognize it. It took me a while to come to the conclusion that I really did want to live." He believed that his illness was an indication that he needed to make some significant life changes. To stay alive, he said, he knew he would have to learn to like himself, restructure his family relationships, and find work that brought him pleasure. This elderly man very rapidly made these changes in his life, changes that usually take years, sometimes a lifetime, of intensive work to accomplish. When I asked him how was this possible, he replied: "It was either change or die. I learn real quick with that kind of stimulus."

But the traditional medical belief that people have little control over their emotional and physical well-being predetermined the research design—and in many ways the results—reported in the NEJM article. The design actually made it impossible to test out what the people in this book have to say: Nothing guarantees survival, but a factor that sets survivors apart may be their ability to change and grow.

THE SEARCH FOR EXTRAORDINARY PATIENTS

Many approaches were used to identify the extraordinary subjects of this book. Physicians in five states were contacted. Most of these doctors were polite and expressed curiosity about the work but explained that they did not have appropriate patients. A few were hostile, calling the project an impossible task or a frivolous venture.

Eventually six physicians, located in different medical facilities, lent their support to the project. They offered the names of potential people to interview, asked colleagues to suggest others, shared background medical information, served as liaison with the medical community when necessary, and even provided facilities for interviewing.

Leads also came from personal acquaintances, newspaper accounts, and magazine articles. But for various reasons it was difficult and sometimes impossible to document the exceptionality of individuals not referred by physicians. Hence they could not be used in this book.

The interviews were open-ended. Since so little is known about this population, the goal was to learn as much as possible about these people and discover how they themselves accounted for their remarkable successes. At the end of the interviews, each person was asked to identify the doctor most familiar with his or her case. These doctors were then contacted and asked to confirm or deny that their patient's course of illness was extraordinary. If possible, they were asked to quantify (using ratios) how unusual they thought the patient's outcome was. Documenting the exceptionality of these subjects followed essentially the same procedure as had been approved by a doctoral dissertation committee when I conducted my doctoral research on the topic.

In every case, a medical authority verified that the person's length of survival was extraordinary. In five cases, a physician specifically labeled the patient's course of illness "a miracle" or a 1-in-1,000 possibility. Detailed medical information was not requested since the physician's judgment was the criterion used to establish exceptionality. The appendix contains the doctors' responses to the questionnaires.

Note that the physicians were asked for their opinions. Assigning probability to medical outcome is somewhat arbitrary, and there is nothing absolute about their estimates. Another physician might assign a higher or lower probability. The point was really to establish that a medical authority felt the patient's progress was extraordinary.

A WORD OF CAUTION

My greatest fear in publishing this work is that it will be used to increase the emotional distance between the seriously ill and the physically healthy. It is commonplace for those of us who are healthy to see the ill, especially the dying, as "other than ourselves." We assume that we are different, that we will not contract some dreaded illness or that, if we do, there is something we will be able to do to overcome it. Distancing from the ill becomes yet another way to avoid confronting the eventuality of our own deaths. However, it is an absolute distortion of the survivors' beliefs to assume that if the very ill person simply tries harder, eats better, visualizes more perfectly, discovers more beauty in life, or develops more spiritually, he or she will be cured.

The limitations of this work are many. Since the emphasis is on survivors, it may seem that "beating" the illness is the only noble outcome. Norman Cousins reminds us that "the tragedy of life is not death but what dies inside us while we live." Many individuals die or remain sick even though they have fully integrated the characteristics described by survivors as life giving. Having an intimate familiarity with many of these people, I do not find the medical successes the most remarkable aspect of their experiences. I am more awed by their resolve to use the disease as an opportunity to find out about their own essence and in the process discover new meaning, joy, and love.

The reader looking for easy answers will not be satisfied. Neither the book nor the individual stories offer prescriptive healing formulas. All the survivors were asked what advice they could offer to people who were faced with a serious illness. Their experience has taught them that in illness, as in life, each must find his or her own way.

An analysis follows each story. As a guide, the analysis may be useful, but it is just one way to understand the experience. The reader is encouraged to undertake his or her own interpretation. Ultimately the only value in presenting these accounts now awaits the meaning you make of them.

RAYMOND BERTÉ

Attitudes themselves have a very potent effect on the immune system. You become different from the person who developed the cancer. Becoming a different personality may change the environment the cancer grew in; it may become so inhospitable that the cancer shrinks.

Michael Lerner,
MacArthur Foundation
"Genius Award" recipient

Contracting cancer is the ordeal of a lifetime. Contracting five different kinds of cancer during the course of one's life seems beyond the scope of human suffering. Raymond Berté has endured—and conquered—five unrelated episodes of cancer. Three of his bouts are discussed here. Perhaps most remarkable is that he can now say, without denying or minimizing his pain, "I do not regret the experience."

Eighteen years ago, a team of specialists discovered that Berté had a very rare form of throat cancer. The treatment of choice was to surgically remove his larynx (voice box). Berté, a professor of rehabilitation counseling, was expected to retire with a permanent disability. Neither college officials nor his doctors believed that he could ever lecture again.

Assisted by a long history of singing and voice lessons, he quickly perfected esophageal speech. Soon he was back at his former position and one of the most sought-after professors at his college.

His struggle with cancer, though, was far from over. Three years later, in 1976, a malignant tumor was discovered between his shoulder blades. A deep hole was cut out of his back, and the tumor was removed. Since the cancer was considered a primary site, Berté was again told not to anticipate any related medical problems.

A year later, Berté detected a lump in the side of his neck. Within a few days, the diagnosis was confirmed—he had cancer for the third time. But now he had cancer of the lymphatic system; surgery could not remove the malignancy.

When I contacted Berté's oncologist, he verified that the medical consensus had been that Raymond would die from the cancer. In fact, Ray was told that he had only six to eighteen months to live. But ten years later he is free of disease and truly alive.

Ray was wearing only a bathing suit when he greeted me at the door of his modernistic farmhouse. Since I knew he was a psychotherapist and college professor, his total lack of formality took me by surprise.

"I'm in the middle of breakfast," he explained. "Why don't you join me on the deck. We can talk and catch some sun." Ray was dark and handsome. His body resembled that of a muscular thirty-five-year-old more than someone of his actual age of fifty-two. Before meeting him, I had concern that I would have difficulty understanding his speech. Though his voice was very deep, with a distinct gravelly sound, the articulation was perfect.

The sundeck offered an expansive view of the countryside. In the distance, a tractor was cutting hay. Ray pointed out an attached studio, where his wife, an artist, was working. Their two children are grown and live on their own.

Ray sat down on a patio chair and reached for the cereal he had been eating. "Do you want something to eat?" he inquired. "Some fruit, perhaps some orange juice?" I told him that after my long trip, juice sounded perfect. To my dismay, Ray leaned over and handed me the glass from which he was drinking.

When my search for extraordinary survivors began nearly eight years ago, I had no idea what personal demons I would have to confront. But now, within three minutes of meeting my first "interviewee," I was face to face with my worst fears about cancer patients—even those who were supposedly cured. Intellectually, of course, I knew that cancer was not contagious. But at some core level, I feared that if I got too close, maybe I could somehow catch his cancer. Without any noticeable delay, I took the glass and forced the juice down.

I think that, at an unconscious level, Raymond was testing me.

Before telling me his story, he needed to know that I could be trusted, for during the next few hours he would lay open the essence of his humanity. Ray began:

In 1972, my dearest friend, who is on the faculty at the University of New Hampshire, asked me to guest lecture for one of his courses. About halfway through my lecture, I started salivating excessively. I had no explanation why it was happening. Then I developed a hoarseness that persisted for a number of weeks. That's when I started having my throat examined. I remember the very first time an ENT [ear, nose, and throat] man examined my throat.

The first thing out of his mouth was, "Well, at least it isn't cancer." I bolted out of my chair; the thought had never entered my mind. I really hadn't thought about cancer as a possibility because I was a nonsmoker, and I'm not a drinker, and those were supposedly considered the two biggest contributing factors. He thought a virus might have settled on the chords. So he put me on an antibiotic.

More than a month later, the problem was still there. It was not painful, but the hoarseness did not go away. I went back and had another doctor in the same office examine my throat. He got all panic stricken. But he wouldn't tell me what his fears were. Then he said, "You have to see the other doctor, but he isn't available at this time." What a shitty thing to do to a patient—communicate a high level of anxiety and then tell the patient he needs to come back later. You're left trying to cope with all that fear.

Finally a third doctor looked at my throat. He told me, "There's a growth in there. Something is going on, and we'll have to do a biopsy on it." So I was booked into the hospital, and the biopsy was performed. It came back negative. Nothing malignant. I was told to continue with the medication, but the hoarseness got progressively worse. After a while longer, the local guy gave up: "I don't know what to do. I suggest that you go to Boston and see the specialist I trained under."

So I went to Boston. The doctor down there, I'll let him remain nameless, said he wanted to do his own biopsy. Again the biopsy came back negative. Now six months have gone by, no definite answers, no real direction. So I check into Mass General Hospital, and they do more and more testing. Finally they came down to it. He told me, "It's malignant, cancer of the throat." There are a lot of hidden areas of the throat that you cannot really see. The biopsies were not picking them up. But they had determined in some way that it was malignant cancer.

After I was in the hospital three or four days, teams of medical people started coming in almost daily. I felt that I was being treated like a piece of protoplasm. Teams of people would enter my room; they would look down my throat, then they would stand back at the foot of my bed and discuss me as if I weren't even present, as if I were a nonhuman. Finally at one point I really got pissed, and I said, "Hey! Nobody's going to look at my throat again. If you're going to talk about me, get the hell out of the room or address me."

Now comes a very significant part of the story, though I did not know it at the time. I was told that the "treatment of choice" was to perform a radical laryngectomy. "We'll cut out your entire larynx and throat and you'll become a laryngectomee. You'll be a neck breather for the rest of your life." I think the insensitive use of terms is atrocious. I could get into that rap for hours.

In a very meek and docile manner, I accepted the diagnosis and the proposed treatment. My throat was cut out.

After the surgery, I was told, "The operation went well, prognosis fine, no metastasis, things should be OK." The other information I got was that there had only been four cases in the history of the medical literature where my particular kind of cancer had settled in the throat. Mine was the first case in thirty years. As a result, my surgeon got calls from all over the world. He lectured about my case in Europe and different parts of the country. I don't say that with any sense of pride. It doesn't mean a goddamn thing to me.

I remember the day they took the bandages off. I'm shaking with fear. The surgeon tells me it looks good. After he leaves, I go to the mirror to look for myself. I'm repulsed by what I see. My Adam's apple is gone, there's a hole where it used to be. I can't stop trembling, as I think, "What's June going to feel." She has such an appreciation of the aesthetic—and I'm ugly as sin.

When I was finally discharged from the hospital, June and I stopped at a restaurant on the Massachusetts Turnpike to have lunch. I ordered some clam chowder that was very hot. I automatically started to blow on it, which began a long silent laugh that turned into a crying jag.

June asked me what was going on. I wrote, "I'm a neck breather now. Do you think it would be improper if I held my spoon up to my stoma in order to blow on my chowder?" Then we both laughed.

The time I was home just waiting for speech therapy to begin was difficult. One day, our eight-year-old daughter went to a lake with some dear friends of ours. She was going to spend the weekend there. But she became sick and stayed in the cottage while the others went off to swim. She grew increasingly ill and called home for help. I was the only one home. The telephone rang and rang and rang. Sensing an urgency in the ringing, I finally picked up the receiver. But, of course, I couldn't talk.

She cried, "Is that you, Dad? Daddy, I'm sick. Daddy, it hurts. I want to come home, Dad. Please!"

I hung up the telephone and jumped in the car, and drove downtown to get June and then to the lake to get my daughter. I never cried so hard in my whole life.

"Benevolently" my doctor had chosen to withhold information from me regarding electroesophageal devices. I didn't know they existed. He thought that if I started using one I wouldn't be motivated to acquire the skill of esophageal speech.

When I went for my next checkup, I had a shiny new Servox (electroesophageal device) hanging on a chord around my neck. My throat surgeon walked in, took one look at the Servox, and said, "What's that?" even though he knew. Answering him, I pressed the instrument to my neck and uttered one of my first words with my new voice: "You son of a bitch. Why didn't you tell me about these?" It really wasn't his decision to make. Had I known about these prostheses from the beginning, I would have been spared a lot of pain.

Soon after the operation, I remember one of the doctors in the medical team asked what I was going to do when I returned home. I wrote that I didn't understand the question. He said, "Obviously you can't go back to teaching. Even if you're lucky enough to learn esophageal speech, it takes two years. And then you can only talk for ten to fifteen minutes at a time since it is so exhausting."

I just don't know what benefit it is for patients to hear *don't, can't, won't.* I think professionals need to appreciate the hypnotic effects their words have on patients. Instead of saying, "if you're lucky enough to," he could have said, "when you learn esophageal speech."

Well, it took me three months to master esophageal speech. Now I regularly lecture for three hours at a time with only a fifteen-minute break.

But when I first returned to Springfield College, I was using an electroesophageal device. I was fearful. Were they listening to anything more than how strange I sounded? I'm sure my nervousness was noticed by the class, and I asked them for reassurance. One by one, the students started yelling out to me: "Keep it coming, Prof." "You sound good to me, Doc." "I hear you loud and clear, Ray." The room was filled with love. When I completed my lecture, the students rose and gave me a standing ovation.

Elizabeth Kübler-Ross says the first significant lesson in her life was that it takes one human being who really cares to make a difference between life and death. On that day, I had a whole classroom.

About three years after my throat operation, my wife and I were sitting on the beach; she turned to me and said, "Gee, Raymond, there's a lump between your shoulder blades. I wonder what it is?" There's an expression that cancer patients use that I think is accurate— once a cancer patient, always a cancer patient. You wonder about every gurgle in your stomach, you question every little pain—could it be cancer? I think almost universally cancer patients know they've got cancer before they are given the diagnosis. There's something in the human psyche that gives you the word.

But, of course, I said to my wife, to allay her fears, "It's probably nothing more than a fatty tissue growth. They're very common, you know. Don't worry about it."

I came back from the beach and went to Michael, a surgeon friend in Springfield. He looked at it, palpated it, and he himself said, "Oh, it's probably nothing. But maybe you should have a surgeon in Boston look at it."

I went to see a Boston surgeon who told me, "We'll take a look at it in three months to see if there's any change in growth and size," you know that kind of bunk. I came back from Boston and thought to myself: What the hell do you do, Ray? How do you live for three months with the possibility it's a growing tumor? So I went back to my surgeon in Springfield. He's a good friend of mine. I said, "Michael, cut that damn thing out. Let's look at it under the scope." So he cut it out, looked at it, and told me it was a malignant tumor. A few days lapsed, and he called me in.

He said, "Well, Ray, I've taken it up with my colleagues, I've discussed it at the tumor conference." They have these tumor conferences every week in major medical centers where doctors get together to discuss their cases and options for treatment. He went on, "The treatment of choice is to cut a piece off between your shoulder blades about yea deep, this wide and this long and get it out of there." Here, you can see. [Ray turned around to show me the very considerable hole in his upper back, now surrounded by extensive muscle development.] For the second time, I accepted the "treatment of choice" without questioning. The high priest had spoken. I accepted the diagnosis, and I submitted to surgery.

After surgery, they told me everything was fine. It was another primary site. They determined that my throat cancer had not metastasized to the back. So I think they got it all again. Fine.

A year or so passes. I discover a lump in the side of my neck. I feel the damn thing. In my mind, I know immediately: "Goddamn it. The cancer has spread." I go to my surgeon. I suggest, "Cut it out, let's take a look at it." So I go outpatient; it's a lymphatic gland. He cuts out about three of them. Of course, I'm awake during this surgery. He holds them in the palm of his hand and says to me, "They look innocent, Ray." I said, "Well, I'll wait and see." And I thought to myself: like hell.

A few days later, I am told these lymphatic glands are cancerous. So now I've got malignant cancer in the lymphatic system. He suggests that I go to another oncologist to do more testing and blah blah blah blah. So I go see this other oncologist; my niece happens to be a nurse in his office. He does some more testing. He did a bone marrow biopsy and gave me the diagnosis. I had fourth-stage bone marrow cancer.

In the diagnosis of cancer, they divide the body up in sections and locations: upper left quadrant, lower right quadrant, upper half, lower half, and so forth. Then the cancer that has been identified is classified in stages. First stage, prognosis excellent. Second stage is obviously more serious. Third stage is deadly. Fourth stage, you're gone.

As a matter of fact, that's what I was told. I was diagnosed terminal. They said make peace with God, because you're not going to be around very long.

I asked, "What are you offering in terms of treatment?"

He said, "Massive chemotherapy and massive radiation."

I looked at him, and I said, "Where is this coming from?"

He replied, "Well, in discussing it with colleagues..." Here it comes for the third time, "'The treatment of choice'..."

That's when I threw up my hands, and I said, "Fuck off!"

"What's wrong?" he wanted to know.

I said, "You know, I've been brought up in a cultural environment that holds the scientific community and the medical profession in great esteem. I haven't lost that. But the difficulty for me is to continue to hear from you that 'the treatment of choice' is... Nobody ever said to me, 'These are some of the options; this is what we think might work; what do you think, Ray?'" I was never involved in any of the decision making.

I said to my doctor, "Steve, from now on I want the best medical information that I can get. And *I* will make the choices!" Very critical.

I reached the conclusion, and this isn't scientific, that somehow or other I was causing my cancer. It was really a wise conclusion for me to reach.

The difficulty for outsiders looking at that statement is that they equate taking responsibility with shame, blame, or guilt. That's not where I'm coming from. I believe that you're either at cause or at effect in this world and in your life. Up to this point in time, I was only accepting the fact that I was at the effect of some power greater than man, the fates, or God, or Yahweh. Well, I stopped believing that and said, "Somehow or other I'm at cause of this. And if I'm at cause, then I can do something about it."

I said to myself, "Now damn it, Ray, you caused it. Now if that's so, and you really believe that, if you caused it—then you can lick it. You can undo what you've caused. You can change that." That's when real critical things started to happen. That's when I began looking at nontraditional methods of treating cancer. That's when I began to research all kinds of topics related to stress, stress management, nutrition, the whole bag.

I began to make critical life changes. At that point my wife and I were thinking about buying this farm. We wanted to get out of the city. Prior to this realization, I said, "What a waste. I'm dying of cancer. What a waste to think about buying a farm and leaving you and the two kids stuck with a mortgage and a big farm."

With my change of attitude and belief—your belief system is critical, if you believe, it works; if you don't believe, it just isn't going to work—I said, "We have to live our life and continue to live it as if I'm going to live to be one hundred years old. We're going to buy the farm." You know we did! We bought this farm. We own all this, as far as you can see.

My diagnosis of terminality carried a lower limit of six months, and the upper limit was eighteen months. Every time I go in now—I go in every three months for a cancer checkup—my oncologist sits there shaking his head, saying, "I don't understand. I don't understand."

Initially there was no support from any medical people for what I was doing. As a matter of fact, I had very little support in my environment, other than a very dear friend, a couple of dear friends, and my wife, who said, "Look, whatever you opt to do, whatever you think is best for you, you know we'll back you on that!" And I needed that.

But everyone else felt that what I was doing was ludicrous. "My God, Ray!" they would say. The nurse working in the oncologist's office was my niece. She would check my records after each appointment. Every time, she'd call me up in tears.

I would talk to the oncologist, and he would say, "Look, if you go for chemotherapy treatment, maybe we can give you three or four more years." And they didn't understand. I'm saying, "Goddamn it, you're talking about giving me three or four more years. That doesn't interest me. I'm not going for three or four more years. I'm talking about beating the rap. [Ray raised his arms and yelled.] I'm going for a WIN!"

That attitude helped keep me alive. In Transactional Analysis terms, it's that spunky little kid inside of you. It's that thrust to life, it's that will to live. It's figuring out ways to survive. Get around it. Go through it or go over it! But you can do it!

Let me give you an example. This guy fell down a flight of stairs.

He was told that he was never going to walk again. Upon learning the medical consensus, he said something interesting: "How the hell can you win a fight if you enter it expecting to lose?" He did something incredible.

He figured that if he could teach himself to move one toe, that would be the beginning. He kept concentrating on his big toe. He focused all of his energy on his big toe. His mother came to visit him one day. He said, "Mother, watch my big toe." He kept saying, "Look at it." He said, "Just keep watching it." And she was watching it. And again he kept saying, "Are you seeing anything?"

She said, "No, I'm not."

"Are you sure?"

She said, "No, I don't see anything."

He said, "Keep watching it, keep watching it."

She says, "I don't see anything moving." But then all of a sudden, she noticed something else. One of his fingers, I think it was his thumb, had started to move. That was the breakthrough. He accomplished what was seemingly impossible. Today this man who was a quadriplegic is out of bed and ambulatory with the use of both arms and legs. That story has a familiar ring. You see, I really wanted to get well.

I'm involved in a great love affair with life. Life has the promise of everything. Death really has the promise of nothing. That's not a denial of life after death or anything of that kind. I do believe that there is a form of existence after we leave this world, and that's a comforting thought. But I want to stay here as long as I can. I love it. I've got too many things to do to leave now.

I always have so damn many things that I want to do, so many projects to accomplish, places to go, people to see. When it comes time to die, I do believe I'll have a sense of completion, a consummation, a Gestalt, or whatever term you wish to use. But I'm still going to feel, damn it, I've got too many things to do.

[Without warning, Ray sprang up from his chair and dashed off into the nearby fields. After a second's hesitation, I chased after him though I had no idea where we were going. Ray was about twenty yards ahead of me when I saw him lunge for his cat. He hit the ground, belly first, arms stretched over his head. But he had the cat, just barely, in his fingertips.

As I caught up, the urgency of the pursuit became apparent. A field mouse was trapped in the cat's jaws. Ray was quick but gentle. He opened the cat's mouth and set the mouse free.

We walked back to the deck without saying a word.]

Since there was no history of cancer in the family tree going back before my parents, even going back to the old country, I did a lot of thinking about how could I possibly contract cancer. In reading Lawrence LeShan's book *You Can Fight for Your Life*, he says he found a consistency in the generation that came to the United States. He suggests that there were probably some cultural influences that lead to cancer in this country that didn't exist in the old country. One of them is stress; nutrition is another part. We are under much more stress, and we also eat very differently than if we were living on a farm in Italy. I'm not talking opinion anymore. It's fact that nutrition has a very important role to play in contributing to cancer, and in getting better, in curing the cancer.

I'm convinced that these were the contributing factors to my getting cancer. One, I did not deal well with stress; I allowed my stress to become distress. Two, my nutritional habits were atrocious. Breakfast was a coffee and a donut. And lunch was a hot dog and a Coke—and everybody knows Coke adds life [laughter].

If I were smart enough, I would have noticed a lot of indicators earlier. As a kid, I had one cold after another. I had impetigo so many times it was embarrassing. Those come from nutritional deficiencies, as far as I'm concerned. I find it fascinating that many people perceive me as being a deviant now, because I choose to eat the way their grandparents ate. They ate fresh fruits and fresh vegetables, no processed foods back then.

I read an article by Albert Schweitzer that greatly impressed me. In studying African tribes, he found that as tribes became more civilized, degenerative diseases began cropping up. In the tribes that remained the most primitive, cancer was almost unheard of, but the ones that became acculturated, or most Americanized, experienced a great proliferation of diseases. Instead of going out and climbing trees to get their food, they started buying canned and processed foods. In addition, I'm sure their stresses increased.

If I was going to live, I needed to deal with stress differently. I discovered my kid time. Your kid time is your fun time, relaxation time. Each person has to determine what it is for himself. For me it is music, a great love of music. Reading. Exercise. Man, I get into my workout. The guys at the health club still can't believe that this is a fifty-two-year-old body.

Once I had cancer, I gave myself permission to do the things I wanted to. Previously I would allow a lot of other things to short-circuit my getting my needs taken care of.

My relationships with everyone that I cared about improved. My sensitivity, my level of awareness, my ability to be with other people just skyrocketed. I made incredible growth in that way.

I'm sure that was healing for me.

I've always had this gift of being able to—it almost sounds jargonny—to empathize with and relate to people. I have great compassion for people. I know that may sound awfully soupy or flowery. That will be etched on my gravestone—I take that back, I'm not going to have a gravestone. I decided my contribution to ecology is to be cremated and to scatter the ashes. But if I were to have a gravestone, one of the words on it would be "compassionate."

When any virtue gets carried to an extreme, I think it becomes a fault. I carried compassion to the point where it became destructive to me. The times I contracted cancer, I found it necessary—mistakenly—to allay everyone else's fears about me and to put them at ease. Instead I should have been dealing more with my own feelings.

One of the things I found absolutely jumping out of people, friends as well as family members, was that because I had cancer, I suddenly made them aware of their own mortality. It scared the hell out of them. Nobody said anything; it was something that I could sense. In rehabilitation counseling, it's what we refer to as the requirement of mourning. People have a need to make those who are ill appear more pathetic and more tragic than they really are in order to bolster their own sense of well-being. If I pick you out to be sicker and more tragic than you are, then I'm better.

One incident really brought that out. Shortly after I got out of the hospital the first time, after I had my throat cut out, I was standing with my wife, my sister, and her husband. It was my sister's anniversary. I saw one of my aunts out of the corner of my eye. The scene is so vivid, oh God, it was sick. She bent over and sidled up to me. She peered up at me like this [Ray imitated a pitiful, forlorn look], looked up in my face, and said, "Is that you, Ray?" I wanted to barf in her face, if I could have on command. It was that "Ooooohhh, poor Ray" scene, devaluing pity. She had a need to

make me out to be a poor suffering bastard in order for her to feel
better and to reassure herself of her own well-being. Weird, but I
saw it a number of times.

Just as these negative feelings can interfere with health, positive
emotions are healing. Humor was very important to me. It's not just
an idea, it has been researched, and there is no question that humor
is healing. Now I see a lot of humor that might have escaped me
previously. I see humor in lots of things.

I can remember the first day they got me out of bed when they
had cut my throat out. In order for me to walk, the intravenous and
other paraphernalia I was hooked up to had to move with me. It
required a nurse on each side of me. At Mass General Hospital,
they have this huge hallway, and it reminded me of a beautiful
running track. I thought, what a great place to run a fifty-yard dash.
Of course, I can't talk, but I'm thinking it. The nurses walked me all
the way to the end of the hall, turned around, and started to bring
me back. But I wasn't ready. I got down in a three-point track stance
and motioned to them, "I'll race you to the other end."

If someone I loved—a friend, a relative, a student—had cancer,
then I would certainly communicate hope and the idea that contracting
cancer, contrary to popular mythology, is not a death sentence.
They need to marshal their own resources, working together with
the best medical information they can get. I think it would be
critical for them to take a look at their diet and their life-style, to
examine how they deal with stress, in particular. It's absolutely
essential that they get vitamin and mineral supplements. From
everything that I have researched, there are certain very important
trace elements, vitamins and minerals that are critical, especially
for cancer patients. I don't think that traditional medicine is going
to work strictly by itself if you don't do these other things.

Most cancer treatment is symptom treatment. You get a tumor,
and they cut it out. The root source of the tumor—why did you
develop the tumor in the first place—remains a mystery. Whatever
the cancer, there's good medical treatment. But it's still symptom
treatment. I think the root causes have to be dealt with.

Finding a physician who "fits" is very important. For my own
treatment, the medical person has to be like me in terms of
openness and flexibility. If I were working with a doctor who

wouldn't cooperate with me on various issues, I would change doctors. I don't want to sound antimedicine, because I'm not. There are some real good medical people out there who don't let their egos get in the way. Those physicians learn from their patients.

[Ray suddenly reached up, snatched a fly in midair, and whacked it on the table. He paused a second. "That's the little Hitler in me."

He paused again, "No, I'm not consistent, but I'm much less uptight about my inconsistency than I used to be."]

The illness was very important; I like me better now.

I don't regret the experience, but it would be a lie to say I wouldn't trade back if I could have my voice again. The reason the experience is so painful to me relates to my singing. I really used to get off on singing. Oh God, I didn't give a damn if anybody else enjoyed it. I used to thrill myself; I'd give myself goosebumps. For twenty years, I studied vocal techniques. Objectively I was really good. They say that a lightbulb shines the brightest just before it burns out. The best singing I ever did in my life was just before I got the throat cancer, and I cannot help but think, had I not contracted the cancer, what I could have accomplished vocally. That is probably the biggest regret. But I can't dwell on that.

There's a reason why I got cancer of the throat—and you won't find this taught in any medical school. The reason has to do with my father. It may sound like I'm reaching awfully deep, but I'm convinced there's a connection there. We really do lay trips on people. We plant seeds that can be very destructive, especially when we say or do things to others when they are most vulnerable. There are studies about organs of susceptibility. If you have been told all your life that you're spineless, you will get cancer of the spine. If you're told that you're a pain in the ass all your life, you get cancer of the anus. My brother never dealt with his bad or negative feelings. He always used to describe them as going right to his stomach. He died of abdominal cancer.

My father would confront me when I was playing with the other children. He would berate the hell out of me in front of all the other kids, "How come you're the only one I can hear. How come you have the biggest mouth on this street?" When he wanted to get my attention from a distance, he would let out a piercing whistle. He'd put those fingers to his mouth, and he'd let out a whistle you could hear for half a mile. It would freeze me in my tracks—talk about a conditioned response—absolutely freeze me in my tracks. I would turn, and he would reach up and grab his own throat like that [Ray put his hands around his neck] and the message was "I'm gonna strangle you! Get your ass over here!" And when I was being led into surgery... [Ray's eyes began to fill. A few minutes passed before he was able to continue.] When I was being led into surgery, I heard a frightened little voice deep inside of me saying, "You won't have to listen to me anymore, Daddy." [Tears began to fall; Ray waited a long time before going on.]

I was with Kübler-Ross when she said there are no coincidences in life. That's a very important belief to me. It's no coincidence that I should get cancer. I don't think I can intellectually make sense out of it, other than to say there's some reason, some purpose to everything. Maybe that power greater than man has a purpose for my getting cancer. It's not that I think He put a finger on me and said, "You're going to get cancer." But perhaps there was the sense that I may be able to make an important contribution. I say that's part of the reason I'm still here. There's a lot I can give people, a lot that I can share. So I say, "Do it!"

My feelings are right on my sleeve. There are no pretenses anymore. When I'm angry you'll know it. If I'm simply displeased, you'll know it. If I'm feeling loving, you'll know it. What I'm thinking, I'll share.

Years ago, I would have covered up, even those feelings about my father. I don't hide my feelings anymore. Whatever people get from me, whatever they see, that's me—good, bad, or indifferent.

OBSERVATIONS

After being diagnosed as terminal, Raymond Berté changed. He changed concrete facets of his life. He moved from the city to the country, a move he had long wanted to make. Even more important were the internal changes. At a time when most individuals would be reeling from the effects of believing that they had lost control of their bodies, Raymond discovered a new personal power and freedom. The stance he took toward his life, that he was responsible for all that happened to him, motivated him to reconstruct his personal relationships, to change his diet, to research information about his cancer, to take charge of his treatment. The responsibility, rather than weighing upon him like a cross to bear, enabled him to begin a "love affair with life." As psychologist Albert Ellis says, "The best years of your life are the ones in which you decide your problems are your own. You don't blame them on your mother, the ecology or the President. You realize that you control your own destiny."

I had heard of Raymond Berté a year before I met him. But what I knew about him had nothing to do with his cancer or extraordinary survival. While working at a mental health center about 100 miles from Raymond's home, I was part of a team interviewing graduate students for the upcoming year. Three students from his college had applied for internships. A standard interview question was: "Describe the most influential teacher in your development as a helper." All three students named Raymond Berte. The interview committee, who had never heard the same teacher cited more than once, listened as these students described the way that Raymond's expectations of excellence had affected their lives. He was said to be compassionate and real, confrontational yet very caring. They said that Raymond had pushed them to their limits to better understand themselves and their motives for wanting to help others.

Raymond is charismatic, in substance as well as style. He puts body and soul into everything, whether it's teaching a class, counseling a cancer patient, or taking a run in the woods. Assertive and powerful, he is a formidable man to contend with. Yet he is not embarrassed to demonstrate his obvious yearning for intimacy. Like his students, I was moved and inspired by this man who gave so much of himself.

Certainly these personal characteristics are not all new developments since the onset of his cancer. But like many other survivors, Raymond made changes so profound that they represented an existential shift. The quality I found most compelling seems to have developed as a result of his trial with cancer: More than any man I have known, Raymond speaks and acts from his heart.

Raymond's will to live is fierce. The decision not to go along passively with the recommended treatment demonstrated his desire to live as well as his willfulness. Raymond refused to collude in a plan that ultimately expected him to die. Raymond was convinced that belief in recovery was essential: "If you believe, it works; if you don't believe, it just isn't going to work." To maintain his hope, he needed to disagree vehemently with anyone, especially a "knowledgeable professional," who was telling him he wouldn't make it. The "fuck off" to his doctor was not an act of defiance nor an expression of denial. He was affirming his own desire and power to stay alive: "When I was diagnosed as terminal, I wouldn't accept it. That's not a denial of reality. It's simply that no expert is going to make a pronouncement of doom on me. If I buy into that, it's the beginning of the end."

More than ten years have passed since Raymond concluded that, since he was responsible for his life and his illness, he would take control of treatment decisions. At the time, such a perspective was considered bizarre and even suicidal. There is growing recognition, however, that living as though one has great power over his or her life actually makes one powerful. Raymond has recently written a book about his laryngectomy: *To Speak Again: Victory over Cancer* (Agawam, Mass.: Phillips Publishing Co., 1987).

Raymond's position is well articulated by some leading business consultants. Dr. Michael Shandler tells his corporate clients, "You are 100 percent responsible for everything that shows up in your life. Other people and the environment have 0 percent responsibility. It does not matter whether or not this statement is true. The question is: Will it be empowering to adopt this 100 percent/0 percent concept of responsibility as an internal psychological stance?"

When asked how or if this concept applies to people who have cancer, Shandler responded:

> It's hard enough to do under normal circumstances—for example, during a fight with your wife—let alone under the stress of serious illness. And, of course, there will be moments of doubting whether your action is the correct action. But anything less than 100 percent responsibility in your operating philosophy can lead to blaming others or justifying your own behavior. If you think that it's up to others or that you can't act until this awful situation changes, the status quo stays intact.

When clients first hear the concept of 100 percent responsibility, some protest, "I don't really have control." In a situation like Raymond's, how can one assume 100 percent responsibility without 100 percent control? Sheldon Kopp, author of *If You Meet the Buddha on the Road, Kill Him!*, offers an uneasy answer: "It may not be fair that a man gets to have total responsibility for his own life without total control over it, but it seems to me that for good or for bad, that's just the way it is."

Seeking out the best medical advice and care available is a critical aspect of assuming responsibility. Raymond used his doctors as consultants. He collected the opinion and advice of experts, seriously weighed their recommendations, and then made his own decisions. Unwilling to be the patient patient, he met with considerable resistance—not just from the medical community, but from friends and relatives who feared his actions were self-destructive.

"It's not enough for your doctor to stop playing God. You've got to get up off your knees," says Marvin Belsky, M.D., author of *How to Choose and Use Your Doctor*. The problem of the disempowered patient is a systems issue—no more caused by doctors than by patients. Doctors have responded to the plea from their patients that they be all-knowing and all-powerful. It seems that we humans want to believe that someone out there really has the answers to the big questions, that someone really is smarter or stronger than we are. The dynamics between psychotherapist and patient, the same dynamics that occur between medical physician and patient, are described by Kopp:

> Certainly at the beginning of treatment, they [the patients] do not imagine for a moment that each of us must save himself. How this experienced inequity between pilgrim and guru comes about is as important as why it occurs. I get to seem so strong and wise as a function of the patient's disowning the responsibility of his own strength and wisdom by projecting these assets onto my not-so-wide shoulders. . . . I am tempted to make the trade . . . [but it] always turns out so badly. . . . I can so easily be fooled that it behooves the patient to pay attention to that possibility.

The way that professional caregivers are trained, especially physicians, fosters authoritarianism. Students learn the "proper" way to interact by imitating the attitudes of their professors and mentors toward them. A system that treats students as though they were children and gives them little respect conveys the message that this is the way to treat others. The education of psychologists, though generally considered less demeaning than what physicians go through, may be hazardous to a person's innate ability to care. One study demonstrated that the ability of students to empathize with others actually declined during the time they were in graduate school learning to become psychologists.

In my own training to become a psychologist, a personally poignant moment came after my course work and internship requirements were completed. I was taking the licensing exam, a rite of passage that legally and symbolically marked the completion of my training status. In the course of this four-hour exam, those who needed to go to the bathroom were always accompanied by a proctor. Three hours into the exam, the line of would-be psychologists waiting to go was very long. When my turn finally came, to speed things up the proctor decided to take two of us at the same time. My fellow student went into the stall first. Once he was finished, I went in. But when I came out, the proctor was gone, having escorted this other fellow back to the exam room. I was left stranded in the bathroom, not sure what the testing officials would do if I were "caught" leaving the bathroom. I was trying to figure out what to do when the chairman of the Licensing Board suddenly walked in. To this day, my only contact with the chairman of the board, a sophisticated man who oversees all psychologists in the state, was to ask, "May I leave the bathroom now?"

Raymond was not concerned that he would feel guilt, blame, or shame if he assumed responsibility for his health but failed to get well. This stance seems consistent with everyday experience: Deep regret swells up from challenges never attempted. People rarely suffer guilt or shame about results if they feel they tried their best.

Ironically, some are inclined to discourage the patient from taking responsibility for fear that he or she will feel guilty if the medical outcome is not successful. Yet few people would advise someone to drop out of a race because of how he might feel if he loses. How many spouses recommend that their partner not go for the promotion because the rejection could be too difficult to bear? Would you tell a friend not to get involved in a new relationship because it may not work out?

A man with acute monocytic and myelocytic leukemia tells of a conversation he had with his physician. He had told his doctor that he had every intention of following the recommended treatment. In addition, he was planning a careful dietary regime, daily meditation, and weekly psychotherapy. His physician, a kindly and well-intended man, said that he was concerned. "If you assume responsibility for your illness, aren't you going to feel guilty if you fail?" he asked. The man with cancer assured his doctor, "If I don't succeed, I'm not going to feel guilty. I'm going to feel dead." By getting involved, there seems little to lose. Feeling responsible for one's life is likely to improve its quality. And it just may lead to action that will be healing.

The concept of patient responsibility, however, can be damaging when it is used inappropriately. Family and friends are often saddened and frightened about the possible death of someone they love. It is not unnatural for them to feel angry with the sick person for "making them" feel that way. But family and friends usually receive far less emotional support than they need, and rather than their communicating their sadness and fear directly, anger may be expressed through an attitude that blames the patient: "She does not really want to get well—otherwise, she would be better by now." That stance is, of course, absurd, but it allows the healthy individual to maintain the illusion that humans really are in control. If death were seen by our society as a natural part of life, blaming the patient for the illness, as well as patient guilt about succumbing to the illness, would never be an issue.

Like many of the survivors I have spoken with, Raymond goes so far as to say he was responsible for contracting his illness. This belief, the precursor to his empowerment, did not lead to guilt or blame. Carl Simonton explains how this is possible. He says, "We develop our diseases for honorable reasons. It's our body's way of telling us that our needs—not just our body's needs but our emotional needs, too—are not being met, and the needs that are fulfilled through our illnesses are important ones."

Others disagree. Harold Benjamin of the Wellness Community, a program whose primary aim is to empower the cancer patient, considers such a stance as troublesome, fraught with the potential of self-blame. I believe the question of whether one's personal habits or emotional state contributed to cancer development is relevant only to the extent that it can be used as a guide for making future changes.

Unfortunately some people will take their cancer as yet another sign that they are inadequate or bad. Failure to get well will be used to symbolically substantiate their worst feelings about themselves. Helping these people understand that their illness does not represent some kind of imperfection in their being is a prerequisite for psychological healing.

When he fell ill, Raymond paid more attention to his own needs and desires. Getting what he needed did not infringe upon the rights of others. In fact, others benefited as a result. The essence of what he desired in his relationships—genuineness, respect, honesty, and caring— is fundamental to all quality human interactions. The challenge and joy he experienced in attempting to create loving relationships was shared by those who engaged in it with him.

Raymond was not delicate in expressing his anger toward others whose feigned caring were attempts to take care of themselves. He resented his aunt's comment, because she was expressing pity, not concern. In *How Can I Help?*, Paul Gorman and Ram Dass make an important distinction. They say that "compassion and pity are very different. Whereas compassion reflects the yearning of the heart to merge and take on some of the suffering, pity is a controlled set of thoughts designed to assure separateness. Compassion is the spontaneous response of love; pity, the involuntary reflex of fear."

Unlike most people, Ray had an intellectual understanding of why certain dynamics, such as the relationship with his aunt, were destructive. But he does not have to filter everything through his intellect before he makes a move. He trusts his raw emotions and uses them as a base of action.

Raymond knows that he needs people who can really be there in the moment. Again, Ram Dass and Gorman discuss why this can be so difficult for the "visitor":

> Instead of being responsive to an actual situation as it is, we come in with our reactions pretaped, just looking for ways to protect them. We may assume people are suffering in ways that they aren't: "Poor baby." "This must be awful for you." "Are you sure you don't want me to call someone?" "Take something for the pain." We wince when someone else gets an injection. We project discomfort onto people about their helplessness which doesn't necessarily exist, or we fail to see the character of the suffering that really is there.

There is a human tendency to place ourselves in the other person's situation, to think how it would feel for us, and then to assume it must be like that for them. But the reality is: We don't really know what the situation would be like for us until we are in it, and someone else may respond differently from us.

Last summer, I met a fourteen-year-old boy for the first time. He had a terminal form of muscular dystrophy, and his physical mobility was progressively deteriorating. He was able to move only a few fingers, with which he controlled his electric wheel chair. I was feeling very bad for this boy who seemed so helpless, so powerless to do anything. At a time when his adult strength should have been emerging, the last vestiges of his life energy were slipping away.

On this warm summer day, we were meeting outside. I felt something flutter along the back of my neck and reflexively flicked it off. It turned out to be a mud hornet who wasn't ready to leave. While I was applying baking soda to my sting, this "helpless" client offered me a glimpse of his perspective. He asked, "Do you want to know why I never get stung?" I said, "Yes." He told me. "When a bee or hornet lands on me, I just sit there."

RELATED RESEARCH

When Dr. Dorothy Smith, a professor at Rutgers University College of Nursing, asked survivors of serious illness, "What do you do to help yourself recover?" what they didn't have to say was perhaps the most significant finding of the study. The researcher discovered that 89 percent of the medical-surgical survivors were surprised even to be asked this question and hesitant to respond. The most common reply was, "I'm doing what the staff tell me to do."

Is the willingness of patients to give up their authority a result of being ill or is the phenomenon more generalized? Stanley Milgram, a professor at Yale University, did a series of experiments that suggest some disturbing answers.

Forty subjects from a wide range of occupations volunteered to be part of an experiment. They were told the study was investigating the effects of punishment on memory. In fact, the researcher was measuring obedience to authority. The subjects were put in charge of administering the punishment to a "learner" (really part of the research team) who was supposedly memorizing material in an adjacent room. The subjects were told to increase the intensity of the electric shock each time the "learner" gave an incorrect answer. A simulated shock generator was used showing thirty voltage levels (ranging from 15 to 450 volts) with written designations from "Slight Shock" to "Danger: Severe Shock."

The researcher reported the preliminary results: "Virtually all subjects, once commanded, went blithely to the end of the board, seemingly indifferent to the verbal designations ('Extreme Shock' and 'Danger: Severe Shock'). This deprived us of an adequate basis for scaling obedient tendencies."

Consequently the researcher decided to introduce protests from the victim, to see at what level subjects would refuse to administer the shocks.

> Starting with 75 volts the learner begins to grunt and moan. At 150 volts he demands to be let out of the experiment. At 180 volts he cries out that he can no longer stand the pain. At 300 volts he refuses to provide any more answers to the memory test, insisting that he is no longer a participant in the experiment and must be freed. In response to this last tactic, the experimenter instructs the naive subject to treat the absence of an answer as equivalent to a wrong answer, and to follow the usual shock procedure. The experimenter reinforces his demand with the statement: "You have no other choice, you must go on!" If the subject refuses to give the next higher level of shock, the experiment is considered at an end.

Milgram describes the results: "To our consternation, even the strongest protest from the victim did not prevent all subjects from administering the harshest punishment." The researcher, who himself was troubled by the findings, concluded: "A substantial proportion of people do what they are told to do, irrespective of the content of the act and without limitations of conscience, so long as they perceive that the command comes from a legitimate authority."

This classic study demonstrates how readily people defer to authority even when they know that authority is asking them to do something wrong. The point is not that traditional medicine is loaded with authoritarian personalities wanting to take over your will. One is just as likely to find this issue among nontraditional healers. Nor is the point that one should not develop a strong dependence on his or her physician. Under many circumstances, such a dependency will be most conducive to healing. Perhaps a reasonable goal to aspire to is that whatever action one takes be done consciously and purposefully.

According to a brochure sponsored by the American Cancer Society, the laryngectomee "cannot lift heavy loads or strain hard because he cannot lock his breath in, as he used to." One of Raymond Berté's physicians gave him still another reason why it would be impossible to work out with weights: "You can't lift weights because when you raise them over your head the clavicles [collarbones] come together and pinch closed your stoma." But Raymond no longer accepted the word from authorities without reflection. By visualizing the activity, he realized that a weightlifter holds the weight over his head for only seconds at a time. Although Raymond had never lifted weights before his operation, weightlifting became important to him afterward. Besides the physiological benefits of the exercise, weightlifting provided visual evidence that he had some real control over his body, its strength, and its appearance.

In general, people who participate in regular exercise tend to have healthier psychological profiles. Exercise reduces stress and depression, both of which are associated with an impaired immune system. A hard workout like Raymond's can raise the body's temperature as much as three degrees above normal. The effect is similar to an acute-phase immune response (that is, the way our bodies respond when we are fighting an infection). Medical researchers think that this response retards the growth of bacteria and viruses. In experiments, rats have been injected with the blood of humans who have exercised for a long period of time. These rats demonstrated the characteristics of an acute immune response—they became feverish, levels of zinc and iron were lowered, and the white blood cell count was elevated.

Scientific evidence suggests a possible link between lack of exercise and cancer. In 1921, two researchers, Silvertsen and Dahlstrom, matched the cause of death and occupations of 86,000 people. Cancer (as a cause of death) was lowest for people who were employed in occupations that demanded the most physical assertion. As Raymond stated, cancer is less prevalent among primitive cultures. Some researchers believe that the decreased levels of physical activity in "advanced" civilization is a contributing factor.

In one experiment, three researchers, Hoffman, Paschkis, and Cantarow, implanted cancerous cells into mice. With one group, they injected an extract from muscle tissues that had been exercised. The other group received an injection of muscle tissue that had not been exercised. The group with the exercised tissue had a decreased rate of cancer growth, and, with a few mice, the cancer actually disappeared.

Carl and Stephanie Simonton, early pioneers in holistic approaches to cancer treatment (their work is further outlined on pages 90 and 91) believe that contrary to popular opinion, many, if not most seriously ill cancer patients, can enjoy normal levels of physical activity. In their research, a majority of subjects—all of whom were considered medically incurable—participated in the same level of activity that they had prior to diagnosis. After consultation with a person's physician, some form of exercise is possible for just about all patients. Some of the Simontons' patients have accomplished quite remarkable physical feats; one person with advanced lung cancer completed a twenty-six-mile marathon.

PHINA DACRI

That which does not kill me, makes me stronger.

Friedrich Nietzsche

I had my first interview with Phina Dacri on her anniversary. Five years before, to the day, her doctor had informed her that she had adenocarcinoma of the lung. In his letter to me, the oncologist wrote, "Her cancer was inoperable because it had metastasized to her chest. The patient was informed that she was incurable."

Phina's oncologist also estimated that the chances were nineteen out of twenty that she would die within three years from the date of diagnosis. Phina beat the odds, but statistics alone cannot convey her uniqueness.

Phina was fifty-seven at that first meeting and had lived all her life in Worcester, Massachusetts. Her father had died five months before she was born. Though the family depended on welfare for its survival, she described her childhood as happy: "We were poor, but anybody could come in and have a piece of bread and butter, whatever we had. My sister used to say, 'I want to give my kids everything I didn't have.' But I always said, 'I want to give my kids what we did have,' because we had closeness."

Phina quit school in the eighth grade to get married. She gave birth to her first child at eighteen and a few years later had another baby. She worked for thirteen years as a winder and doffer at a local mill. For the next twenty-five years, she was employed as a cashier at Woolworth's and then Grant's. Before leaving, she had worked her way up to head cashier, overseeing twenty others.

In her polyester jumpsuit and running shoes, Phina projected constant motion. The rapidity of her speech matched the image. In fact, six hours of interviews with her produced more typed transcript than other interviews twice as long. Her words seemed driven by a special vitality and sense of urgency. She was a woman determined to live each moment fully.

Her conversational style bordered on stream of consciousness, and she appeared not to censor, nor need to censor, her statements, however intimate or revealing. At the end of the interview, she thanked me for the opportunity to share her complete story at last and possibly help others who were sick.

Emotionally Phina was open and uninhibited. She shed a tear as she discussed her poor marital relationship and smiled when she spoke of all the children who wanted her to get well. Though our interview was conducted in a vacant room of an oncology unit at a city hospital, she was as relaxed as if she were talking with a friend at her own kitchen table.

You want to hear something I did the other night? I told the doctor and he says, "Oh, you're crazy, Phina." I went to bed and I wheeze a lot, and I was going, "cHAW cHAW cHAW cHAW," like a cackle, so I says that's the death rattle. I got up and I wrote a letter to my son. I says, "I've been happy, more than ever. Nobody is to blame for anything. You've been a good boy, and I love you." The next morning, I was still alive so I tore the letter up! [Phina laughed.]

I don't like anybody having guilt when I'm gone, I don't want them to feel sad for anything they did to me. Hey, it's forgotten. Well, maybe not with my son-in-law, but forgiven anyway.

My daughter and her husband asked us to move into their house, into their apartment. My husband said we shouldn't go, and we shouldn't have. After we moved in, my son-in-law says, "You're going to be treated like tenants." And it started right away, rent increases $10, then $20 every year.

I was there one day when my daughter come home with the baby.

My daughter was kind of crying, and I said, "Gee, Ken, she's upset." He said, "Out!" Just like that. And I went out. He kicked me out. I went home crying all the way. It was hard. My husband said he would never go back, but I went back for more and more.

Now it's different. I can be my own person, where before I always had to hold back, wondering, "Will it hurt them? Will I cause trouble?" Life was all rules: "You can't do this. You can do that." Now I do what I want, when I want.

If anybody hurts me now, they know point blank. Like years ago, if my son-in-law or daughter-in-law hurt me, I wouldn't say nothing. Today I'll tell 'em. If they like it, OK; if they don't, OK. Hey, they respect me more.

At first, I don't think my family liked the independence. Like the other day, my daughter said to me, "Boy, you're awfully strong." I wasn't sure if she was saying, "That's good" or that it was a crime. I am an independent person. Maybe there's a little stubbornness in there, too: I'll show you I can do it. I think that attitude does help a lot with any sickness.

I've always been proud. I told my sister, if she comes to the hospital and sees that I'm dying, then her job is to pluck the hairs from my chin if they start growing! [Phina laughed.] I told my son, I said, "If you come and see me and I'm dying, you sit outside. Come in every hour and say 'hi,' but don't sit and watch me go." I don't want anybody looking at me while I go. I even made out a will 'cause when I go, I don't want anybody yelling at Chris. All he has to do is show the will. I let him know where this is or that is. He used to get mad at me, but now he understands.

I'm not afraid to go, but I'm not ready. I have plenty to live for. I'm not a world traveler, it's the small things I want to live for. I want to live for my family, my grandchildren. I laugh: Before I wanted to see my grandchildren get big, now they're big, the oldest is eighteen. So now I want to see them get married. After I see them get married, I want to see their first child. You know, I'm gonna be impossible to get rid of! Every year, there's going to be something I want to see. I want to see my first great grandchild. I want to be a great-grandmother, then I want to be a great-great-grandmother. I'm grabbing, and the day is gonna come, but I'm not gonna die from cancer. I'll die like everybody else, from...pneumonia. That's it.

My daughter laughs: I renewed a magazine for five years 'cause it was cheaper. She says, "Boy, do you have confidence." It's true. Deep down I think I knew I was going to get better even though I made all the arrangements.

But I wasn't always like this. I remember when they told me. I was in the hospital with angina.

They had put me in the year before. I was a new patient of Dr. Russell's, that's when he says to me nicely, "Phina, would you quit smoking?" If he said, "You gotta," I never would have. But he just hit me the right way. I didn't even have a last cigarette, I quit.

Then I says to him, "You know what's going to happen, my lungs are going to clear out and then they'll find something else."

Well, the next year I start getting these chest pains, and I think I'm having a heart attack. My husband dropped me off at the emergency room; he worries so much about his car, it's only a '73. He says, "Do you mind if I go park the car first?" I says, "You mean you can't walk me in?" That's what he thinks of his car. It's metal, you can get a new one of those, but a new human being you don't get so easy.

This was at the beginning, so those things don't help; but I didn't let it get me down. I thought that I was a little better than a car. This is the first time I'm wallowing up at all 'cause that was a sore spot.

So he's out parking his car while they admit me and start treating me like a heart attack. I don't see him again until I'm in my room.

Dr. Russell comes in. They put me on the fifth floor, and I hate that room 'cause that's where they had to tell me. I think it was five twenty-five. I always said I never wanted to be told if I have cancer, but I never said it to my doctor. He said, "Phina, there's something on your lung, and we believe it's malignant." He said it right out. I could see the tears roll down him, he was crying. I held it in while he was there. It was the worst day of my life. After he left, the girl that was in there with me—we became good friends—we cried and cried and cried. I cried the whole day.

They were going to take a biopsy and they did and it was. I think I cried once more after that, but that's about it. I never got depressed; I don't understand. My famous saying is, "I was too stupid to get scared."

God put me in a shock, and I hope the hell I stay there the rest of my life, 'cause it's beautiful. I think I felt good because my kids were set; they were married, I didn't have all those big worries. If I had little kids at home, it probably would've been different.

My son is thirty-six, and she's forty. It's funny nobody broke down when they heard. I know they felt real bad, but I don't think they realized what cancer was, maybe because I was never laid up. I mean I never had pain until after the radiation. My son always said he would do anything he could for me. With the children or grandchildren, I mention it like candy; I say "cancer" just like I say I'm going for a walk. I brought it out in the open, and that's good.

But my husband, I don't mean he's heartless, but he's not the type that can give you much. I never felt like I could talk about it at home. If I talked about the cancer, he'd get all worried like he had it or something. So when I said anything he'd look at me like I was going on and on and on.

But I will not let him get me down, and he knows it. No matter what he does. I have a fusion, cancer, degenerative arthritis, gall bladder, and my neck—I have to hang from the door to relieve it, and if he thinks he's gonna get me down after all that, nope, I'm sorry.

If I let him get me down that would have been it. Before I would cry over it, but now maybe I cry once a month. When I do, you wouldn't believe it. I cry and I say, "What are you crying for? Your eyes are going to be sore tomorrow," and I stop. Honestly.

It's changed so much. If he gets mad, like I'm sorry, you know what I mean, but life is too short. Imagine how I'd feel if I had a beautiful—[Phina chuckled]—heh-heh—relationship, God, I'd be on cloud nine. I'm half way there now, but with a good relationship it'd be a lot better.

In the beginning, I'd lay on the couch with the pillows around me, and if I wanted something I'd never say will you get me this or that. I'd roll off the couch and I'd go get it. Part of it was stubbornness and part of it was not wanting to hear him go, "Blah, blah, blah." I'd always make supper. You find a way to do what you have to.

I wanted to get well; I didn't want to be laid up. It was the same when I had my fusion. I was in a great big barrel of a thing, up to about here [shoulder height]. You can't bend over, but I'm stubborn. I used to get on my hands and knees to make the bed, and tuck it in as I went around.

Like the difference between my husband and I, he's got a kink in his back and he can't do nothing. Now I've got the world's worst back. You just keep going, that's all. If you sit and worry and brood, it don't get you nowhere. Now he's saying he can't eat. He lost seventeen pounds worrying about not eating. It was nothing. I don't say, "Oh God, what's gonna happen tomorrow?" If it's there tomorrow, I can cry. If I start crying, I'll say, "Don't let me cry; my eyes will just burn in the morning." I'll say, "God, please, I want to sleep now. So tomorrow morning, whatever you think should come." I blame Him for everything; believe me it's beautiful, if people could just live that way. So I go to sleep instead of crying.

The illness changed my life more than anything else could have. When you're getting close to death, every minute counts. When you're breathing, you have everything that counts. I do everything I want to now. If everybody could just live like that. It's beautiful.

I was a very nervous person before. I was terrible. I used to worry about everything, every little thing. If I thought my daughter was mad, I'd be nervous. I don't do any of that now. Don't get me wrong: It doesn't all go away; I mean a little bit will stay, but I won't waste the time like I did before. I'll find something else to get my mind off it.

Now I give all my worries to God. It makes a beautiful cop-out. I don't have to worry about it. He's taking care of it.

I became a born-again Christian after the cancer.

I think you have to have faith. When I went through the cancer, I did get faith. I get right down on my knees, and I say, "I'm leaving it in your hands," and that's it. I will assure you: If you don't believe, it isn't going to work. I'm sure He has listened to me, listened to me plenty.

Ya know how they touch you, the priest, and ya fall. Well, I watched some on TV and I laughed, because I think the priest pushed 'em. One day I was sitting there, the priest went by and touched me, and I went out on the chair. I got slain. It must be that I wanted it so bad, that it happened. It's the faith.

If something worries me, I throw it all in God's hands or the doctor's hands. I never ask my doctors questions. I put all my faith in them, and I think that's an important part of my story.

I'll never ask another question, because I did after I had the cancer about two months. Everybody said I should ask questions. So

I said to Dr. Sherman, "How come they call lung cancer the killer disease?"

And he says, "'Cause lung cancer is the worst. Ninety percent die."

And I said, "Well, I could have lived my whole life without knowing that." Then I said, "Well, my girlfriend had it, and they operated. How come you didn't operate on me?"

He says, "'Cause you have it in your chest, too."

I says, "I could have lived my whole life without knowing that either." But then I figure, well, she's dead now, so maybe it's not so bad they can't operate.

I didn't know it was the worst when they told me I had cancer. I mentally blocked it; I didn't want to know then. Some of those things you don't have to know, so I don't ask any more questions. What they tell me to do, I do.

I was prepared to die at first, and I figured in six to eight months I'm gone. The first two or three months, I was positive I was gonna die. I never said any of this to anybody. But I'm saying this to you.

Every time I came to see Dr. Sherman, he made me feel better. When I went to the clinic, they would open the door, and it wasn't like I was going to get treated for cancer. It was like I was going to see some people. They're very, very good here. It's not dreary. They treat you just like a person, do you know what I mean? They never brush me off in here. You come in, and here you're Mrs. Dacri. Here you are friends. It's like we're next-door neighbors.

I have two wonderful doctors, Dr. Sherman and Dr. Russell. Your doctor means the world.

They don't pull any punches, but they're good about it. They don't raise my hope by saying, "You're gonna get better." But Dr. Sherman all the way through would say, "Boy, you're doing beeeautiful, but I can't promise..." which is true.

He gave me the hope because when he started telling me about the treatment, he put down a two- or three-year plan. So I figure maybe I got a little bit of time.

So he gave me the start, and that was the important part. Never did make me feel like I was gonna die there.

We always talked ahead. We never talked death; we never used the word, and that helped a lot. At first, he kept saying, "Come back next month." I figured, "Hey, I got another month. Great. I'll grab everything I can get." Then it was three months. Now it's every year, just for precaution.

Faith is the important part. Like I said, they started me off on that road. They have a unit down at the University Medical School where they prepare you to die. If they put me on that unit then, I'd know I'm dying. I think that could do you in. Really, I never got panicked. I was concerned; believe me, I was concerned. But when you get down to it, I think I always knew that I could lick it. I knew the responsibility was mine.

Dr. Sherman takes away the fear. You go in, right away he shakes your hand. "How ya been?" You talk your family, he talks his family, and then you forget what you're even there for. I always wanted a doctor-patient relationship.

We have become very good friends over the years, and I'm sure he's like that with everybody. I know a lot who have gone to him, and they love him. When I first went to him, I think there were thirteen or fourteen of us. Now they're all gone.

The poor doctor. I feel so bad for Dr. Sherman because he sees a lot die. It must be very rewarding to see a few walking around. You don't see too many miracles. And I probably am. A walking miracle. Last time I saw Dr. Sherman, he and Dr. Russell are joking and they're saying, "You know, you're not supposed to be around."

Between them all, they had an awful lot of compassion. Dr. Russell and Dr. Sherman really take this cancer bit to heart.

I always call Dr. Russell a nosy doctor, lovingly though, because he finds everything. Now he's working on a gall bladder problem with me. He's a young fellow, very dedicated, you don't find many like him. Do you know what Dr. Russell did to me one day? I almost passed out. I had told him how Dr. Sherman saw something that he wanted to look into harder. Well, two days later, the phone rang, it was Dr. Russell, he wanted to know how I was making out. I said, "Gee, you made my day. No doctor ever called me up and was worried about me. I never got a call from a doctor in all my life."

They are as proud of me as can be. Like when Dr. Sherman called me up and said that you wanted to talk with me, I said to my daughter, "Dr. Sherman probably wants me because he hasn't got any more living patients. He wants me because I'm the last one alive."

There's some reason I was left here. God kept me around for

something. When Dr. Sherman called about talking to you, I said, "Gee, maybe that's why." If I could talk to people with cancer I'd tell 'em, "Don't worry too much." It's an awfully hard thing to do but, boy, that can kill you. I would tell them, "Don't look at dying as death, look to life."

God left me here for some purpose, and someday I gotta find out why.

The second interview with Phina was conducted five years after the first. I met her at her new home, a subsidized high-rise apartment for the elderly. We greeted each other, not as old friends, but with the memory that we had once shared the most intimate of conversations. The fact that we could meet again confirmed the belief that there had been meaning in the first discussion.

Although it was Tuesday, with no holidays in sight, her home was filled with the smell of a roasting turkey. In her kitchen, many of the regular Thanksgiving fixings were in some stage of preparation. She explained that she had picked up a turkey cheap. She thought it would be fun to invite five or six of her elderly neighbors over for dinner while she was at it.

Before the interview began, we each had some old business to take care of. I was curious to find out if any researchers had contacted her since my last visit. It had been ten years now since Phina was first diagnosed with terminal cancer, and there was no doubt that she was an extraordinary survivor worthy of study. When she said no, I asked if that didn't surprise her. She explained, "No. It's the same with the news. They like to give you the ugly."

Her question for me confirmed how involved she had been in the first interview, working hard to make her own sense of the experience. She wanted to know if I could remember asking, "Did you believe you were going to lick the illness?" She then told me, "You hit it on the head. Because I think I always knew I could do it."

Since I could not remember the specifics, I went back and listened to the old recording. Different from her usual quick response in the rest of that interview, there was a pause before she answered my question: "You know, deep down I think that's what kept me here. I've never even thought of that before. In the back of my mind, son of a gun, I must have figured yes, I am going to get better."

Phina then told me about some of the major changes in her life since we last met:

One day I got up and I said to myself, "Since God let you live, I don't think he meant you to be a drudger. He didn't mean you should live like this." So I made a whole new turnover. I got this place here sight unseen. The lady in charge asked, "Don't you want to see it first?"

I said, "I'll take it anyway." Now it's like I was born here. I am able to be myself here.

My husband didn't think I would go through with it.

The lawyer said to me, "You sure, after forty-one years, you want to do this?"

I says, "I'm positive. I can't take it." I don't think God brought me through the cancer to be a jerk. He's not letting me stay here to take all that baloney. God isn't like that. In other words, I had to pay Him back for what He did for me.

Oh, it's hard, I needed to and I was scared, but the illnesses wouldn't keep me back.

I could barely talk to my husband about them. When I had broken the vertebrae, I would moan and groan at night, but he'd never come in and say, "You all right?"

About two weeks before I went to the lawyer's, it was real cold. Nobody could start their car. And my husband couldn't. So I says to him, "Maybe it's the battery." But he called the garage, and he told them, "Pick up the car and put in everything new that it needs." Now this is a '73 car we're talking about; it's not a Rolls-Royce.

My daughter told me that he used the house money. That got me so bad that I hit the wall, packed three bags, and I left. I stayed for two nights at the Holiday Inn.

In the weeks I was trying to decide what to do, my husband never once talked to me.

The day I was going for the divorce, I knelt down and I said, "Please, God, give me an inkling in the morning that I'm doing right."

The next morning I got up, and I says something and my husband goes, "Yak yak yak."

"Thank you, God. I'm going." It was both Good Friday and April Fool's Day the day we got divorced.

Some people think marriage is a fifty-fifty split. I don't believe that, because some people can give better than others. I love doing for people. So I would gladly give 90 percent if I got 10. But I didn't.

I'll only get married again when someone makes my heart go thump thump thump thump. But I'm not going to iron, I'm not going to sew, I'm not going to cook, so who's going to marry me? I'm not going back—this life is too good. I love it. I love it. I love it. I've never been happier.

Oh, I've got a lot of problems, but I don't dwell on them. I've been trying to volunteer, so I called the American Cancer Society to see about typing with one finger. I thought they could drop some stuff off here for me to type. But they said no. I can't make regular days to go because I got Epstein Barr syndrome since last time. Some days I'm flat on my back sleeping the whole day.

I figure I can take anything but just don't cut my tongue out, because then I won't have anything to live for. I'd want to die. Now I'm a big mouth; I used to be awfully shy.

When I had the cancer, I wanted a group because I couldn't talk about my cancer at home. But there were no cancer groups, so I joined Weight Watchers. I needed to talk to people and I needed to lose weight, so I figured what the heck.

I was 118 all my life, but then with the cancer I went to 183. Everybody else loses weight with cancer. Not me. I've talked to people with EB virus. They all knew they had it because they were losing weight. But I never lose weight with anything.

I love to eat. When I was in the hospital with the cancer, this girl and I would order two suppers and keep one for late at night. You don't know how fat you're getting until you go home. My doctor used to get mad at me because I was worried about getting fat. It's funny, if you're close to death, you'd think you would say, "What the hell, I'm gonna eat." But I always worried. If there was any chance that I was gonna get better, what am I gonna do if I have to go home and lose a hundred pounds first?

I had a picture taken back then with Dr. Sherman. I said a couple of years ago, "Can I have the fat picture?" He says, "Only if you take another one."

It took me a year and a half to lose fifty-three pounds, but we had a ball. I did away with my favorite sweets, and I tried to get the grease out of everything. But this was to lose weight, not for my cancer.

I think those group things are beautiful. I used to be very shy before the cancer. I can speak my mind much better now. Like the other day, I went down to Honey Farms with my girlfriend. I had six bottles of Slice to return. She says, "We don't sell that kind of Slice."

I says, "Well, the Slice people'd be glad to take any kind." She goes, "Blah blah blah," really carrying on, but she took it.

Then I says, "Can I have a lottery ticket?"

She gets all sarcastic. "Well, what kind do you want?"

I finally says to her, "My God, how can you stay with the public?"

Then my girlfriend says to her, "Are you working alone?"

I says, "Well, who can work with her?"

She says to me, "I don't need you."

And I said, "Don't worry, you're not going to have me."

I can't stand that. When you're with the public, you can't be like that. I know many times when I worked at Woolworth's or Grant's I hated the person, but I had that smile.

Since I speak my mind better, my relationships have changed. My daughter and I will get a few uppy words, and then all of a sudden we catch ourselves; we explain ourselves to each other, and we know where we stand. Before we would go weeks, and I used to fester. But no, I can't do that anymore. I don't have time for that anymore.

Oh, don't get me wrong, I have my days. My sister-in-law just died with cancer of the lungs and brain. I've had an awful lot of deaths this year. I lost my brother. It gets to you, but he was down to a skeleton; the stroke was a blessing really because all he wanted to do was to stay in bed.

I lost my best pal, my nephew. That was the hardest. When I got the divorce, he's the first one that said, "I'm here for ya." We went to the cemetery, and he dropped dead as soon as we came home.

Every year he and I would go to all the graves. We thought we were standing at his father's grave, so we planted flowers and prayed for him there. We laughed when we found out we were at the wrong grave. We always had a ball together.

When we got to his house after the cemetery, he must've been starting to feel bad 'cause he said, "Gee, Auntie, you're a pest, you're giving me an anxiety attack." We laughed. I remember he stooped over and I said, "Gee Rick, what a big fat cooler you got"; it showed all his bum-bum. When I got home they said Ricky had a very bad heart attack. He died right in front of his nine-year-old. The doctors said he died before he hit the ground.

I mean we've been through it, but somehow things work out. I have a sister who likes me and a sister who don't. Now the one who don't, died. That was Ricky's mother. The day she died, she called me up. I just got out of the shower, and I was dripping wet. I had the towel around me, but she was talking so nice I couldn't hang up on her. I knew we were getting close.

She never used to come to the cemetery with Ricky and me to plant flowers. But the day he died, she called up Ricky. He said, "If you be good to Auntie, you can come." So she got to be with her son on his last day.

I have a feeling that when you die you go up there. It's this nice big place where everyone is friends. I'm going to be with my mother, but she'll be Helen, not my mother, and Ricky will be Ricky; it won't be nephew and aunt.

You're all friends when you go up there, and you're all happy together.

But you're not going to meet your family, because no way would God put my sister up there and let her see the way Ricky's wife is acting down here—running around, neglecting the kids. You think God's going to let her watch that? No way is God going to punish you like that. When you die, you're supposed to be peaceful.

As for me, I'm not afraid to go, but I'm not ready. I love life, I love it, I love every bit of it. Since all of this cancer stuff happened, I found myself as a person. I do like myself now. I love myself. And if you don't love yourself, you can't love anyone else. I'm damn proud of myself. I am, I'm damn proud of myself. Every year they find something new, this year it was the Epstein Barr virus. And if they don't find something next year, I'll probably be disappointed. Each time they find something new, it just makes me stronger.

My life is beautiful now. I used to wake up and say, "Ho hum, another day." Now I wake up and say, "Thank you, God."

OBSERVATIONS

When Albert Einstein was asked, "What is the most important question facing human beings?" he replied, "Is the Universe friendly?"

Phina Dacri's universe is a very friendly one. The power in control of her life on earth—God—is loving and beneficent. She finds no reason to fear even death since God would only construct an afterlife consistent with His ultimate compassion.

God's will is for Phina to find a life of meaning, happiness, and health. If Phina can successfully align herself with His will, if she can let go and leave everything in His hands, her fulfillment is assured. Phina's devotion to a God who resides in heaven, to a God who wants her to discover her full potential, is a devotion to herself.

Her desire to put everything in His hands may sound passive and abnegating of responsibility, but, in fact, her effort to accomplish this is a difficult and disciplined process. Letting go of one's ego for what one knows to be a higher truth requires conviction of purpose and faith. There is paradox in Phina's situation: In order to succeed, she has had to be very responsible about letting go of responsibility. One time, she put it this way: "I'm working harder than I ever did before. Like before, if I went into a store, and they give me an extra five dollars, I'd say, 'Great, I'm ahead by five.' But now I wouldn't take it. You know I said I'm working harder, but in another way I'm really not. I'm putting it all in somebody else's hands. At the same time, I'm doing my part."

Before her cancer, she was willing to stay in a marriage that brought pain and despair. But her obligation to God was to honor herself and to honor her gift of life. Thus, at a time when most people would hold on more tightly than ever (after forty years of marriage, financial difficulties, multiple illnesses, and uncertainty about whether or not she was going to die), Phina initiated a separation and divorce.

On the day of her court appearance, she asked God for a sign that the dissolution of her marriage was necessary. A psychological interpretation is that she projected her own unconscious desires onto some other all-knowing being. "God" acted as an intermediary, providing direct access to her inner needs and desires. The answers she got, then, were really from her own inner core. Since her inner self (like all of ours) is all loving and all knowing, does it matter if the message came from her inner godliness or from a God external to her own being?

Unlike most people who initiate a divorce, Phina's pain was not deepened by self-doubts. She was saddened over what she had to do, but she experienced neither indecision with its usual companion, depression, nor guilt about her actions. Her direct communion with God did more than allow her to end a relationship that was destructive to her well-being. It became essential to do so. "I don't think God brought me through the cancer to be a jerk." Though she treated her marital relationship with sanctity, her commitment to God and God's will took precedence over any other vows she had made.

There are many physicians, philosophers, and spiritual teachers, as well as the miraculously cured, who think that faith like hers is absolutely healing. Placebo studies demonstrate the power of one's belief to heal (see page 197). And in *Love, Medicine & Miracles*, Bernie Siegel tells about a patient with advanced pancreatic cancer who went home to die. When she reappeared at the office months later—cured—she was asked what had happened. Her explanation was uncannily similar to Phina's: "I decided to live to be a hundred and leave my troubles to God." Siegel's experience with cancer patients has convinced him that "this peace of mind can heal anything. I believe faith is the essence, a simple solution, yet too hard for most people to practice."

Comparing a radiation oncology unit with heaven may seem unimaginable, yet Phina described them in remarkably similar terms. She depicted heaven as a nice big place in the sky where "you're all friends and you're all happy together." The view may be a bit concrete for some, but the absence of barriers between people does suggest a universal ideal. In her oncology unit, as in heaven, the barriers that keep people distant from one another are insignificant: "Here you are friends. It's like we're next-door neighbors." The doctor talks his family, and she talks her family. She feels cared about because of who she is, not because of her disease.

In some important ways, Phina's feeling for her two physicians was similar to her feeling for God. More than once, she mentioned God and her doctors in the same breath and was direct about the significance of her relationship with them: "Your doctor means the world." Unselfconsciously, she informed us that she "put all her faith in her doctors." In fact, it seemed that the only reason she asked them any questions at all was because of pressure from others to do so; and since she wasn't acting on her own initiative, it was not surprising that she would have preferred it if they hadn't answered her.

Her orientation, then, seems diametrically opposed to the emerging new view of the "responsible patient." Phina's story is a wonderful reminder that a single path will not serve everyone. It is also important to note that, given the qualities of her two primary physicians, her trust in them did not appear naive or misplaced. They were skilled and knowledgeable practitioners. In addition, as mature human beings, they felt genuine concern for her well-being, celebrating in her successes and empathizing with her life pain.

According to Norman Cousins, "the central question to be asked about hospitals—or about doctors for that matter—is whether they inspire the patient with the confidence that he or she is in the right place; whether they enable him to have trust in those who seek to heal him; in short, whether he has the expectation that good things will happen." Phina's experience with Dr. Sherman was consistently positive: "Every time I came to see Dr. Sherman, he made me feel better." His style and manner helped to maximize her feelings of hope. Again, Cousins indicates the emotional and medical value of a physician's "bedside manner":

> Being able to diagnose correctly is a good test of medical competence. Being able to tell the patient what he or she has to know is a good test of medical artistry. . . . Is it possible to communicate negative information in such a way that it is received by the patient as a challenge rather than as a death sentence? The issue here is not whether to tell the truth but how to tell the truth. Truth can be told in a way that can potentiate a patient or devastate him. It can lead to challenge or set the stage for shattering defeat.

Over the years, I have interviewed a number of Dr. Sherman's cancer patients. Their responses are consistent. He has a remarkable ability to put the cards on the table without making any illness, however serious, seem hopeless. In Phina's case, for example, he let her know that she should get her affairs in order, yet the underlying message he transmitted, by detailing a long-term treatment plan, was that he expected her to be around for a long time.

Curious to better understand this life-giving skill, I interviewed Dr.

Sherman. I wanted to know the origin of his ability to engender hope in patients even while he fully disclosed the statistical bleakness of their prognoses. I asked him if this wisdom was learned from a mentor or perhaps an especially enlightened course in medical school. No such examples came to mind.

Weeks following our interview, we were casually talking, sharing childhood stories. He let me know that as a child he was (and technically still is) severely dyslexic. In the fourth, fifth, and sixth grades, school officials told him and his parents how incapacitating his learning disability was. He would never be on a college track, they said. Perhaps he might eventually be able to learn a manual trade. After earning a BA from McGill University, graduating from Boston University Medical School, and completing a residency at Harvard Medical School, the power of hope has become far more than an abstraction for this doctor.

In the past, Phina presented a front to others that betrayed her true emotions. She constantly wore a smile for the years she worked at Woolworth's or Grant's, even when dealing with customers she hated. Phina's metaphor—"I used to fester"—may actually describe the way in which her bottled-up emotions undermined her physical well-being.

Popular films present many examples of how this kind of self-betrayal can destroy health. Woody Allen's character in *Manhattan* tells us, "I don't get mad, I grow tumors." In *Doctor Zhivago*, a character says:

> Your health is bound to be affected, if, day after day, you say the opposite of what you feel, if you grovel before what you dislike and rejoice at what brings you nothing but misfortune. Our nervous system isn't just a fiction; it's a part of our physical body, and our soul exists in space, and is inside us, like the teeth in our mouth. It can't be forever violated with impunity.

After developing cancer, Phina changed in ways that allowed her to be more true to herself. She made changes in her life situation that were very concrete. Equally important were the internal changes she made in the way she felt about herself. For the first time, she experienced self-love. It became easier to share her true feelings with others as she grew more confident about her basic goodness.

Liking herself, loving herself, she had less reason to be on guard. She opened herself to the many forms of beauty and joy in her life. More receptive to all that life had to offer, she had more reason to stay alive.

Phina's changed outlook on life may or may not have influenced her recovery. It certainly eased her physical pain. Her various illnesses and complications are usually associated with significant pain and discomfort. Frequently they incapacitate the individual. Yet Phina moved through life with a vigor that is rare for even a healthy person.

Martin Buber tells the story of a Hasidic Rabbi who was plagued with long-standing pain:

> From youth until old age Rabbi Yitzhak Eisik suffered from an ailment which was known to involve very great pain. His physician once asked him how he managed to endure such pain without complaining or groaning. He replied: "You would understand that readily enough if you thought of the pain as scrubbing and soaking the soul in a strong solution. Since this is so, one cannot do otherwise than accept such pain with love and not grumble. After a time, one gains the strength to endure the present pain. It is always only the question of a moment, for the pain which has passed is no longer present, and who would be so foolish as to concern himself with future pain!"

Phina, too, did not suffer over anticipatory pain: "I don't say, 'Oh God, what's gonna happen tomorrow?' If it's there tomorrow, I can cry." Her contract with God wisely included a provision that exempted her from worry about future pain: "I'll say 'God, please, I want to sleep now. So tomorrow morning, whatever you think should come.' ... So I go to sleep instead of crying."

Phina's approach achieved the same results as those taught by pain control experts. For example, Dr. Jon Kabat-Zinn, an associate professor of medicine, encourages pain patients to dispassionately observe the sensations of pain. Similar to Phina's relationship to her pain, the individual is taught to accept the sensations for what they are, without fearing what they might become or without attaching any symbolic significance. For example, the patient stops fearing that "my pain will become unbearable" and stops believing that "I am suffering from pain because I did something wrong and deserve it." Generally, when a person can do this, he or she will experience less suffering.

RELATED RESEARCH

According to the cancer personality theory, the "typical" person who develops cancer is likely to have an inadequate outlet for his or her emotions, especially anger. If there is any truth to this theory, an important question presents itself: Can expressing emotions affect a malignancy? Dr. Lydia Temshok of the University of California studied individuals with melanoma. She compared the rate of tumor growth for patients who more openly expressed their feelings with patients who were more suppressed. As part of the study, the researcher asked the patients to discuss a time in their recent past when they were angry. Their responses indicated how varied the sample was: "Some said they could not remember ever being angry, while others got right into it, even gritting their teeth and smashing the table." The study, published in the *Journal of Psychosomatic Research*, found that those who more openly expressed their emotions had a lower rate of cell division and more lymphocytes. Both were observable factors suggesting that the emotionally expressive group would have a more favorable course of illness.

Other researchers report related findings. Leonard Derogatis, Ph.D., and Martin Abeloff, Ph.D., concluded that woman with metastatic breast cancer who expressed their hostility survived longer than nonassertive, compliant woman.

Intuitively we may think that Phina's joy translates into not just a higher quality of life, but a longer life as well. Recent scientific findings support the intuition. For seven years, Dr. Sandra Levy studied a group of women with advanced breast cancer. She found that the patients' levels of joy could actually predict how long they would live. In fact, the number of sites of metastasis (the number of places the cancer had spread to) was a less useful predictor of survival than how joyful the person was.

It is important to mention that we are presumably talking about genuine levels of joy. Trying to appear happy for others when the patient is not feeling that way is destructive; it separates the ill person from his true feelings and makes him feel distant from others. Similarly, the friend or relative who tells the patient how he ought to feel, that he needs to be happy, is not acting in the best interest of the person who is ill. A doctoral study by Dr. Mark Raymond Otis at the University of Florida actually found that positive affect was negatively related to outcome for lung cancer patients.

In my own counseling with cancer patients, I become concerned when a person suffers a serious loss, especially divorce or the death of someone whom they loved. My experience has demonstrated, and research is corroborative, that loss can impede the functioning of the immune system. A breakthrough study in this area was conducted in Australia in 1977. Dr. R. W. Bartrop and his associates gave blood tests to men and women whose spouses had very recently died. The first blood tests, conducted just two weeks after the partner's death, were not significantly different from normal. In another four weeks, however, blood tests indicated that the subjects' immune systems were depressed. The report, published in *Lancet*, concluded, "This is the first time severe psychological stress has been shown to produce a measurable abnormality in immune function which is not obviously caused by hormonal changes."

In a follow-up study, Dr. Steven Schleifer and his associates from the Mount Sinai School of Medicine in New York examined the effect of grief on men. Their sample group consisted of men whose wives were terminally ill. The researchers compared the responsiveness of the husbands' immune systems before and after their wives died. Two months after the death of their spouses, the responsiveness of the husbands' immune systems were significantly lowered. Gradually functioning improved, but even after a year the immunopotency for some men was still less than it had been prior to their wives' deaths.

Phina experienced multiple losses in the five years between the first interview and the second, a time when she was at risk of recurrence. Her brother and sister died, a nephew who was also one of her best friends died, and she was divorced. Though the losses were great, she did not suffer a setback from the cancer, nor was she overwhelmed with grief, as research theory might suggest.

But research deals with reactions to loss that are typical ones. Anytime we assume that an individual will fit the statistic, we underestimate and devalue very real human differences. In fact, some losses, such as the termination of an unhappy marriage or the end of a troubled sibling relationship, may actually be healing.

To understand Phina's experience, it is essential to recognize how very friendly her universe is. She lives her life with a working appreciation of the big picture. From such a vantage point, life circumstances—even death—are not likely to be devastating. For everything is unfolding just the way it is supposed to.

NORMAN COUSINS

This is the true joy in life, the being used for a purpose recognized by yourself as a right one; the being thoroughly worn out before you are thrown on the scrap heap; the being a force of Nature instead of a feverish selfish little clod of ailments and grievances-complaining that the world will not devote itself to making you happy.

George Bernard Shaw

In 1964, Norman Cousins was stricken with ankylosing spondylitis, a devastating collagen disease characterized by disintegration of the spine. The likelihood of recovery was approximately one in five hundred, according to specialists.

After submitting to standard medical procedures for a brief time, Cousins devised his own treatment plan. Against the advice of medical opinion, he discharged himself from the hospital and checked into a hotel. Laughter was his treatment of choice. The nurse he hired played Marx Brothers films and Candid Camera clips, and read aloud from various humor books. In addition, after researching the therapeutic benefits of vitamin C, he chose to take huge doses of the vitamin intravenously. Despite the prediction of expert medical personnel, his recovery was practically total.

Best known for his forty years at the helm of the *Saturday Review*, Cousins also carried out international peace missions for United States presidents and other world leaders. At the request of Pope John XXIII, he helped win the freedom of Catholic cardinals imprisoned in Eastern Europe. Today he is the leading spokesman working to bridge the perceived gap between "scientific" and "holistic" medical approaches.

Long before Norman Cousins ever contracted a serious illness, he had
come in touch with his own potency in the world. Unlike most patients,
Cousins maintained and even nurtured his sense of personal power once
ill. Now he seeks to empower others:

> When I work with patients I prove to them that they have
> far greater powers than they realize. I demonstrate this by
> showing them that they have the ability to move their blood
> around. I lead them step-by-step as they move their blood
> around and finally I have them move the blood to their hands.
> When they see that they have the power to increase the surface
> temperature of their skin by 10 degrees or more, their relation-
> ship to their bodies and to their illness changes.
> Once you liberate patients from helplessness, freeing them
> from the depression that helplessness produces is only a short
> step away. Depression is a very specific factor impairing the
> immune system. Consequently, by freeing patients from de-
> pression, we've been able to show that there's an almost
> automatic boost in the production of disease-fighting cells.

In the following interview, Cousins discusses his exceptional progress
with a very serious heart attack. Drawing upon his successful fight with
ankylosing spondylitis and vast medical knowledge, Cousins created a
new unorthodox treatment formula. Once again, his remarkable course
of recovery defied the most expert medical predictions.

Bill Hitzig, Cousins's physician, compared his patient's recovery to
the recovery that was so celebrated in *Anatomy of an Illness*. He said,
"His 1980 heart attack was even more serious than the illness from
which he recovered in 1964, and his present recovery, I believe, is even
more remarkable than the recovery from his previous illness."

[Mr. Cousins begins his story by describing his life-style prior to the
illness:]

My heart attack was really coming to me. I had been traveling all
over the world, battling the time zones, battling sleeplessness. There
were regular stresses in getting from place to place, having to
scramble across the country to make engagements, and then not

always making them. I found myself drawn into a schedule beyond human endurance.

The heart attack was a very severe one. An enzyme count that measures the amount of muscle destruction demonstrated the heart attack was several times more severe than average. Fortunately, I did have enough previous experience to eliminate the most serious threats to my survival.

I have always felt that the reason most patients with heart attacks never reach the hospital alive is that the panic produced by the heart attack can be as serious as the disease itself. Panic may be the factor that pushes the heart beyond its tolerance level. Panic produces a type of flooding that further destabilizes the heart and that constricts the blood vessels. So the heart, which is already in a precarious state, has to try to pump blood through the narrowed openings, creating an additional, intolerable burden.

I had been telling my students [at the UCLA School of Medicine] all along that, with heart attacks, you have two problems, two threats. One is represented by the disease itself; the other is represented by the panic. If you can control the panic, you are in a much better position to control the disease. The propensity of illness to produce a chain reaction in which the panic intensifies the illness, the illness intensifies the pain, the pain intensifies the panic, and so on, is one of the unhappiest aspects of serious illness.

First, you must liberate the patient from the panic. Having drummed that into medical students and myself, when the heart attack came, I knew that my chances would be improved if I could eliminate the panic.

We keep an oxygen tank, a small one, around the house for the same reason we keep a fire extinguisher—it is a good thing to have in an emergency. Consequently, when the attack occurred, I could direct my wife in hooking me up, so I knew that my heart was getting the oxygen it needed.

When the paramedics arrived, I could keep them at bay, and I could be spared their heroics. On the ride to the hospital, I had them turn off the siren and the clanger, and had them slow down, because the ride inside an ambulance, in one of those careening vehicles, with the sirens going is really as panic-producing as any experience in this world.

When I arrived at the hospital, the dean of the medical school and other medical personnel were waiting for me. They were scared. For I also had congestive heart failure, I was bringing up blood, and I had severe left ventricular dysfunction. Despite these facts, I was absolutely confident. I could reassure them and tell them that they were looking at the damndest healing machine that had ever been wheeled into the hospital. Having committed myself to that, I was going to prove it.

The doctors would call my absolute confidence denial, but it can be beneficial to deny, to defy the verdict you think is attached to the diagnosis. If you can recognize that the diagnosis is a challenge, not a verdict, and that there are resources to work with, and not all of them lie outside yourself, you can liberate the body from the complicating factors caused by fear. It seems to me that this frees the healing system—whatever that is—to assert itself and also creates an environment in which medical treatment can do its best.

I think it is important for physicians to be a little humble and say that they don't know enough to make predictions in any given case. Avoiding language that stifles hope gives patients a chance to breathe spiritually.

My confidence enabled me to dispense with the lysine and the morphine that are usually necessary to bridge the emergency, but you pay a price for them.

I know that the disease represents a breakdown in the human body's healing system. Medication is only a crude approximation of what the body is supposed to do for itself. Panic, fear, and depression inhibit the ability of the body's own apothecary to function properly. I was attempting to rely on what the real, ultimate truths in medicine are. The modalities in medicine change. The way you treated ulcers five years ago is entirely different from the way you treat them today. Yet you expect people to subscribe to the new methodology. The one thing that remains constant is what goes on inside the body itself.

I refused the treatment that the doctors said was absolutely urgent. They wanted to give me heart surgery. They said that I could not survive without it. I was told that the amount of heart muscle destruction was so great that I did not have the reserve to function normally, and that I could be totalled at almost any point.

Helplessness is a product of our education; we seem to be convinced that serious illness always proceeds in a straight line unless interrupted by some outside agencies. It's a kind of education that prepares us for weakness rather than strength. We're not educated in the essential robustness of the human body. Consequently victory seems to be very elusive.

I can recall the precise moment when I knew I was going to make it. That moment came during a conversation with my cardiologist. He told me that I needed surgery because my arteries were clogged. I asked, "Is this irreversible?" He said, "Quite definitely, the situation is irreversible by itself." The moment he said that, I could feel a great surge of energy. I could not restrain my face from breaking out into a smile. He asked, "Did I say anything funny?" I said, "No, Stuart, I'm just saying to myself, 'Here we go again.'"

The term "irreversible" really set off a fire inside me. I can still feel the terrific surge. There's a certain amount of joy that comes from knowing that you're going to win no matter what may be involved.

I must confess that I was excited about the entire experience. My excitement began with the notion of irreversibility: I knew that I might not be able to unclog my arteries but I could develop compensatory circulation inside the heart.

Yet I felt that what my cardiologist did was absolutely essential— he had to make me understand what I was up against. I wanted to make my decision on the basis of all the facts, and I did not want those facts prettified. I also appreciate the fact that my cardiologist did not try to make me appear stupid. He was not angry. He may not agree with me, but he respected what I had to say.

In the hospital, I was not encouraged by some people to be as active as I was. My family doctor was terribly concerned. He himself had had a heart attack, not as severe as mine, but it was severe enough. He laid down the law to me. He did not want me to write—I was writing a play at the time. He did not want me to get all that excitement, all that fatigue. He did not even want me to read. He did not want me to brush my own teeth. With his heart attack, he had to be absolutely motionless for almost six weeks. But I never agreed with that therapy.

After the heart attack, he flew out to see me. When he came into my room, I sat up in bed. He shook his finger, "Hey, don't do that!" He also advised me not to laugh. Apparently he felt that I was right when I said [in *Anatomy of an Illness*] that laughter was a form of internal jogging. On the day after my heart attack, he called me up and warned me against the sort of thing I did before—especially laughter.

After this conversation, my wife came into the hospital room, and I asked her to read the morning newspaper to me. She came across an account of an editor of a newspaper not far from L.A. feuding with a city councilman. He had referred to the city councilman as a "Greek orator." The councilman protested, saying that he regarded this to be an ethnic slur. A reporter from the *Los Angeles Times* called up the editor and said, "Are you going to apologize?" The editor replied, "Certainly not. I was just being a little ambiguous. Actually, I should have said he's a loquacious asshole." I burst out laughing, and I knew that laughter was still my friend. I've been laughing ever since.

Humor has been healing for me, but I would not suggest what I did for everybody. I do not think it would work for everyone.

This brings us to a basic principle, namely, that the statistical approach to illness cannot be regarded as absolute. To some extent, every individual places his or her own stamp on the disease. The wise physician recognizes the extent to which this is true and acts accordingly. The physician has to listen. The physician has to talk. The physician has to engage. Unfortunately too many physicians just talk these days; they're not paid to listen. Medicaid and Medi-CAL pay according to technology and the tests that are performed, so the physician is forced to a stand that is inimical to the patient's welfare.

For the first six months after my heart attack, I did not go to the office at all. I would go out on a walking track twice a day. At first, I would have to sit down after walking sixty yards. At night, I would get a little breathless, and with the slightest exertion I would have arrhythmias. I knew that healing the heart was an ongoing process. It takes some time, and I was ready to invest as much time as was necessary. I worked my way up to six miles a day. I also had to bring down my cholesterol level. My wife values good nutrition, and she relished the opportunity to make nutrition basic in our lives. I brought my cholesterol down from 285 to 170 with diet and the fun I was having.

All along, my wife was certain that I would recover. She is

absolutely impervious to intimations of disaster. For example, when I was commuting back in the East, we would rush to try to make the train. If we were too late, she would say, "We'll get it at the next station." And she would go off in pursuit of the train. When we would get to the next station, if they had already pulled out, she would say, "We'll get it at the next station." And off we'd go. Of course, we drove all the way into New York that way.

She doesn't give up. And it would be impossible for her to believe that anything that happened to me was irreversible.

I was lucky. No one argued with me to try to push me in a different direction. I could very easily have had a wife prone to hysteria crying, "Oh, Norm, the cardiologist says you're not going to make it if you don't do this. Oh, you've got to do it, Norman, you've got to do it. Please do what the doctor says. Do what the doctor says."

Instead, my wife said, "Go to it!" She really believed it, too. She wasn't just trying to back me up. She had lived with me long enough to know that I was right.

The knowledge that people cared—my wife, family, friends—meant a great deal to me. It was important to my recovery. On a scale of 1 to 100, it would be 101. I must say that the outpouring of cards and letters was extremely nourishing.

But I didn't want to see everybody. Not because I was antisocial but because to me the biggest capital in life is time. It's a question of balance—I wanted to make the most of this experience.

My illness solidified the meaningful relationships and made the marginal relationships more marginal. It brought me closer to my friends, I guess, because I was able to spend more time with them.

I was also able to play more golf. The year after my heart attack, I was designated the most improved player of the year at the golf course. I took six strokes off my handicap.

I am playing golf again, I am now playing tennis again, I am traveling again. My heart is doing all the things it's not supposed to be able to do.

I have slowed down in ways in which I had to slow down, and speeded up in ways in which I could afford to speed up. As an example, three weeks ago I looked at the schedule for the latter part of June and July. There were items on the schedule that I wanted very much to do. I was invited to address the special session on

disarmament of the United Nations. I was chairman of the delega-
tion of the American Writers that was sent to meet with leading
Soviet writers in Moscow; I had board meetings of the Kettering
Foundation and the Mott Foundation. I just wiped them all clean. I
could not have done that before the heart attack. The reason I did
that was not because I didn't think that I could take it, but because I
felt that I would flourish without those commitments.

The illness changed the threshold of my conscience. Previously I
could not have taken off every Thursday night to play golf as I do
now. And I do it with the greatest of ease, without the slightest
twinge of conscience. I no longer live an unrequited life with
respect to the things that I want to do.

I don't regret my illnesses. I don't think that God was unkind to
me. I don't think that I was deprived of anything. Obviously I would
not have objected if I had been spared both those experiences, but
having had them, I learned something, I derived a great deal of
energy from it, and was able, I think, as a consequence to reach a
new plateau in life.

This is a pretty big universe we are in. No one has been able to
calculate the amount of light-years that is involved in traversing from
one end to the other, if there is such a thing as one end to the other, or
around the whole, if there is such a thing as being able to go around
the whole. Infinity is a rather remarkable concept. In contemplating
this vast infinity, the ultimate truth I arrive at is that the highest prize the
universe has to offer is human life. And, possessed of this gift of life, I
am not going to relinquish it unless I really have to.

OBSERVATIONS

After interviewing Norman Cousins on two separate occasions, I knew
that his sense of self-possession was remarkable, his integrity beyond
doubt. Nevertheless, I found myself wondering, could his recollection
of events during the crisis be accurate? After all, he had suffered a
massive heart attack with congestive heart failure; sudden coronary
death was an imminent possibility, and with his extensive medical
background, he doubtless was aware of the danger involved.

The literature concerned with the psychology of fear is straightfor-

ward. A "fight or flight" response (which, in addition to other physiological changes, places an increased load on the heart) is the natural
human response to danger. Three physicians confirm, however, that
contrary to the way people usually react in the midst of a life-
threatening medical crisis, Cousins remained calm and even managed to
stay in control. Dr. Omar Fareed wrote in *The Healing Heart*:

> Imagine the scene in the emergency room of the UCLA
> Hospital. Dean Sherman Mellinkoff, of the UCLA School of
> Medicine, and several of the school's top cardiologists are
> awaiting the arrival by ambulance of a patient who has just
> had a heart attack. The telephoned report from the paramedics
> is alarming; it says that the patient is coughing up blood, an
> ominous indication of congestive heart failure. The swinging
> doors to the emergency room open wide and a rolling stretcher
> comes through. The patient sits up, waves, grins, and says,
> "Gentlemen, I want you to know that you're looking at the
> darnedest healing machine that's ever been wheeled into this
> hospital."

Cousins's remarkable attitude during the medical crisis continued
during the rehabilitation. He would do everything possible to maximize
his chances of survival. Sacrifices were necessary, of course, but his
commitment to health never preempted his commitment to a rich and
full life. In fact, savoring life's pleasures was just as fundamental to the
treatment program he developed as exercise and diet.

The approach was unorthodox but never reckless. He carefully
weighed all the available medical information before making any major
decisions. Some of the decisions might have placed him in medical
jeopardy, for his interpretation of the scientific facts was not the sole
criterion for decision making. Any action had to be compatible with his
deeply held values. Cousins's doctors asked him to be more cautious;
even when they didn't agree with a decision, they respected his
determination to make the quality of life a top priority. After learning
that he had resumed his strenuous tennis playing, David S. Cannom, a
cardiologist and colleague of Cousins, said, "It is probably just as well
that I am not there to see it, for I should probably risk a heart attack
myself just to observe someone running at top speed who had congestive
heart failure only recently." This physician went on to say, "No

cardiologist can say, given the massiveness of the heart attack, that he is no longer at risk from another attack or even sudden death. What I do know is that he functions superbly in every way that is vital to him and that . . . he is getting the most and the best out of whatever may be possible.''

Cousins obviously came into the illness with personal and institutional resources far greater than those of the average patient. He possessed significant knowledge of the human body in general and heart disease in particular. His confidence in the basic vitality of the human body—a conviction that fights against any serious illness—had been tested and fortified by his successful battle with ankylosing spondylitis many years before. His professional network included some of the most renowned physicians in the world. These personal relationships did more than guarantee that he would receive the best medical care available. His celebrity status and the respect his doctors felt for him gave him extraordinary latitude to be himself without the prospect of ridicule or derision. Another patient who bolts upright and refers to himself as the ''darnedest healing machine'' might be labeled psychotic. One physician attributed Cousins's decision to forego the bypass surgery and refuse the angiogram to the ''keen sense of the integrity of his body''; similar action by another patient might be dismissed as massive denial.

Although Cousins's resources and experience were far from ordinary, there are everyday implications. His composure and sense of humor while struggling for his very life may seem heroic, but a little planning can minimize the trauma of most medical emergencies. When an emergency procedure is established and known by all family members— with important telephone numbers close to the phone—the person under siege is comforted by the knowledge that his or her primary needs are taken care of. It may sound exotic, but those who run the risk of an emergency requiring oxygen can learn how to administer it with a doctor's prescription and a little instruction. And though only the rarest of patients finds himself confronted with an illness that he once lectured medical students about, everyone reading this book can seek out and understand the medical basis of his or her illness and the rationale for treatment.

There are important lessons to be learned from his experience, but the message is not to imitate Cousins's behavior. In fact, he was perhaps the first influential spokesman, steeped in a scientific tradition, to communicate that "every individual places his or her own stamp on the disease." When Cousins wrote *Anatomy of an Illness*, he intended a metaphorical interpretation of laughter. Laughter was a symbol for the therapeutic value of all positive emotions. Some people, however, adopted his story as a prescriptive formula for healing: Laughter was the panacea that could be made to fit any situation.

A colleague of mine tells about a young man who sought therapy because he was emotionally distraught and physically ill. While still a newlywed, his wife had unexpectedly died following a very brief illness. A few months after his wife's death, he determined it was time to stop his grieving. Continued mourning, he told himself, was a waste, a needless self-indulgence. He thought it was time to get on with his life. Learning of Cousins's "laughter cure," he spent many hours reading joke books and watching funny movies. Like Cousins, he even checked out Marx Brothers movies and footage from Candid Camera. After several months of this laughter regimen, the young man developed a peptic ulcer, severely disturbed sleep patterns, and a very poor appetite.

His attempts to coerce his emotions into responding as he thought they ought to was exacting its toll. In this man's case, crying was far more essential than laughing. He recovered only after he found the courage to express feelings that were painful but his own.

Anatomy of an Illness was the first book of its kind to generate significant interest among medical professionals and discover, as well, a large and responsive lay audience. Cousins's anecdotal account, backed by research available at the time (1979), presented a strong scientific argument for the connection between emotions and health. Since then, thousands of additional studies have proven beyond question the existence of this relationship. Researchers are now concerned with identifying the extent of the connection and the specific variables involved.

One line of inquiry concerns research into multiple personalities, a rare psychiatric illness. In the case of multiple personality disorder, two or more distinct personalities exist within the same person, and the individual's behavior may vary dramatically depending upon the personality in charge at any given time. Investigations have shown that a single individual with multiple personalities can actually possess different physical characteristics, depending upon the particular personality that is dominating. Even qualities that are subject to objective measurements, such as brain wave patterns and curvature of the cornea, vary within the same person according to the predominant personality.

In an article published in the *American Journal of Clinical Hypnosis*, Dr. Bennett Braun described the case of a man who had an allergic reaction to citrus juices—he would itch, develop a rash, and blister—when one of his personalities was in control but had no reaction when another one was. In a second case, Braun presented a woman who was "deathly allergic to cats" when one of her personalities was dominant. In a different personality, however, "she could sit and play with a cat for considerable periods of time, even be scratched and licked by the cat, without any apparent allergic response." Another study of multiple personalities documented the account of a woman whose diabetes was very difficult to treat. The disease and her insulin requirements fluctuated depending upon which personality was in control. A third study reported the case of a man who was color blind in one personality but had normal color vision in another.

Research such as this cannot prove whether or not emotions affect a particular individual's recovery. However, like Cousins's experience, such studies corroborate the powerful connection between mind and body.

JOE GODINSKI

> Creativity is my life. If I deny that in any way I'm killing a part of myself.
>
> **Joe Godinski**

After an especially virulent form of cancer was discovered in Joe Godinski's lungs, medical experts said he would die shortly. The medical predictions were backed by the authority of statistics collected from thousands of similar cases. A physician wrote this about Joe's course of illness:

> Once the patient was diagnosed with lung cancer (oat cell), he had one lobe of his left lung removed, received radiation, and refused chemotherapy. A year later, he developed a brain metastasis, which was treated with radiation. When he developed a tumor behind his right eye, he was treated again with radiation. The likelihood that Joe could survive for even one year was approximately one in a thousand.

Joe has had no trace of cancer for more than a decade. His complete cure is established. The physician also stated, "His healing is by any standard a miracle."

Joe Godinski and I had arranged to meet in front of the Washington Monument. I had neglected to get a physical description of him, but,

71

recognizing our mutual anticipation, we spotted each other easily. From the medical report, I knew that he was forty-five and, given his history with cancer, I was expecting an old forty-five. I'm not sure if it was the soft yet steady bounce in his step or the unwrinkled facial skin, but Joe actually appeared far younger than his age.

After shaking hands, he asked if I had eaten breakfast yet, though it was about one o'clock in the afternoon. As we walked, Joe explained that since his gig the night before had run very late, he was just getting up. As he guided me to a large cafeteria-style deli, I was curious to see what Joe would eat. He was only the fourth person I had interviewed, but some patterns among the interviewees were emerging. The most apparent was that they each had made radical changes and were now eating primarily "health foods." We went to the counter to order: Bacon, eggs, white toast with butter and jelly, and coffee with two sugars was breakfast for him. A chocolate chip cookie and another coffee was dessert.

As I set up my microphone and tape recorder in this busy and very noisy restaurant, I did not know if it would be possible to conduct the interview. But the overly solicitous waitress, the din of background voices, even the young couple fighting next to us were only minor distractions.

My total absorption had just as much to do with Joe's style as the drama he was unfolding. Clearly Joe's words were not part of a rehearsed talk. In fact, I found myself wondering if he had ever revealed his entire story before, for, most of the time, it seemed that he had little idea what would come out next. But he was obviously ready to share himself, and the history that accompanied him without pretense or defense. Joe began:

Even now, when I think about this experience, it gives me the willies. I was playing the piano in the parlor. My mother and a girlfriend of hers were downstairs in the sitting room. All of a sudden, for some reason or other, I started laughing. I want to tell you, this laugh came from my very bowels. It was so deep, once I started laughing I couldn't stop. I didn't know what I was laughing at, but I continued to laugh, and I couldn't stop. I was rolling all over the floor. After a few minutes, my mother and her friend came charging up. They thought there was something wrong with me.

When they realized I was laughing, they probably figured I was a little strange, but they just went back downstairs. I continued laughing.

It was a tremendous gutsy, get-it-all-out-through-laughing experience. To this day, I don't know what I was laughing at, but the thought passed through my mind, "What a tremendous joke this all is." Everything. I realized then: There's absolutely nothing wrong with me—which was really the first time I felt that way.

Those are the kinds of things that did it for me, that healed me.

I always thought there was a lot wrong with me. I was taught that as a child. Sometimes you meet people who are so lucky. You can see that they've been loved all their lives. They've been told they are great and encouraged to take chances. Since they've been loved, they know what love is. It's beautiful. I envy that. I wish it had happened to me. But it didn't.

I don't think I really understand what love is. Intellectually I understand, but I don't really know what the feeling is.

And yet I had this healing experience that is really about love in a very intimate and personal way. So I know love deeply, but in a general way. I haven't known those most intense feelings with just one other person. I mean I love the world, I love humanity. I'm just not sure how I feel about people. [Joe laughed.]

My parents were divorced when I was very young. My father took my brother. My mother brought my sister and me to New York City. She had no job or anything. I was three years old, and my sister was ten. We went to this Catholic boarding school, and it was a nightmare.

There was a nun in charge of the school who was a real prick. She loved inflicting pain and giving orders. She beat the hell out of us. There's no doubt about that.

When I was six, I graduated into the "big boys" group. That's when a lot of the abuse happened. I was very much a rebel when I was a kid. I got the worst of it because I refused to knuckle under. But the more I tried not to give in, the more she hurt me. This head nun used to punch me and beat the hell out of me and then kick me when I was down. Her favorite thing was to grab my muscles under here [Joe held his underarm] and dig her fingernails in, and just squeeze. It was abuse. I was abused, no doubt about it.

I've since met four or five other kids who went to the same school. They're all screwed up from it, too.

There was nobody to stop it. When you're a kid, you're just afraid of it. I didn't say anything to my mother. Now as an adult I can say that was really ridiculous, not to say anything, but what do you know as a kid? I mean I must've deserved it; adults, especially nuns wouldn't whack you around unless you deserve it. [Joe laughed.]

I reached the conclusion that there must be something wrong with me, that I'm bad news—everybody leaves me. My father went away, my mother hardly ever comes to see me, and I'm getting beat up by a nun. This was really the seed of my cancer.

I went to the school when I was about four and stayed there 'til I was seven or eight. Then I came out for a year, but my mother sent me back because I was misbehaving; she said I wasn't cooperating at home. I think I was nine when I came out.

So that really set the stage for the way my life went. I believed all that stuff about myself, and so I felt shitty about myself for many, many years. I grew up hating everybody and everything.

After so many years, the body stores the messages you've been giving yourself, and the body doesn't let go easily. I mean you have to be a superhuman being to get that stuff out of you, to get rid of it. It's such a monumental task, maybe one in twelve million can attempt it. Therapy is one way, but it just seems so inefficient.

Even today I have a lot of work to do. I'm not ready to be really open with other people yet. I was healed, but I'm no guru. I'm fearful. I'm anxious. Eventually, I know it'll be great. But it's a bitch to change, it really is.

[Joe had just finished breakfast, when he asked, "Do you mind if I smoke?" I laughed, certain he was spoofing the couple next to us, who were both smoking after their meal. Since he continued to wait for my answer, I knew he was serious. I told him I didn't understand. He explained:]

My cancer was not environmentally caused. Smoking had nothing to do with my getting cancer; the source was emotional. If the source had been environmental, the solution would have been entirely different. There are certain things that I have to take care of. Smoking is one of them. Unlike other people I've heard about, I really didn't become more sensitive to my body. I really did nothing. No diet, no exercise. I chew my food a lot better now; that's really the only difference. I eat very slowly and chew my food very well. But no special diets. As you can see, maybe I should lose a few pounds. But I love eating. My mother is the greatest cook in the world. It's wonderful. I'm very passionate about food.

Growing up, I think I saw my father once when I was seven or eight. I didn't see him for a very long time after that. In college, summertimes, I used to go up to see him. He had a business, and I'd help him out. But they weren't pleasant times. He had a great sense of humor, but he sure didn't know how to be with his children.

My brother didn't benefit from him. He went through an awful lot of tough times with him. My brother and I never used to talk; now, suddenly, after my illness we became very close.

We're like night and day, couldn't be more dissimilar. I could tell you what he does, maybe that'll tell you something: He's been working in the service for eighteen years. He doesn't know who I am or what I want. He's not an artistic fellow or sensitive in those ways. But he's a very generous and loving person.

In my family, I seem to be the only one who's artistic, interested in the aesthetic, or ever questioned aloud about life. There was nobody, no cousins, no uncles, that I could talk to. Or, if there were, they certainly hid it very well.

So growing up I always felt very separated from everyone else. Because of the sensitivity and because I was hit and abused emotionally, I couldn't get a hold of myself, so I was not able to connect with anyone else.

I couldn't appreciate my difference, my creativity, my interest in music and art. I suffered with it. I hated being different. All my life, until the cancer, I've been fighting against my difference.

When I was struggling as a kid, and even as an adult, I was never disciplined with my music. I wanted to play but I'd always do something to sabotage it. I'd study piano for a year, then I'd lay off for two, and then study for six months, then lay off for a year. I was never focused.

Now I've been practicing every day for more than three years. I enjoy it, so I do it. Playing is so much more satisfying than before. I love music. That's what sustains me.

Before I got sick I didn't realize to what extent creativity was important to me. But now I know that creativity is my life. If I deny that in any way, I'm killing a part of myself. My willingness to go ahead and use it probably helped a lot in the healing process. It continues to help.

When I was thirty-two, after many, many odd jobs and the service, I tried to get serious about my music. I left New York for Valencia, California. I was going to study electronic music at the Disney School.

To pay for school, I applied for my VA benefits. I had at least a couple of thousand dollars coming to me. But for some reason I never received the money, so I was at the school through the graces of a professor. Students complained once they learned I was there gratis. I had to leave.

Once I left school, I had to make a living. So I sold encyclopedias. The first year worked out pretty well; the second and third years got progressively worse. I mean selling encyclopedias, going door to door, that's not me. It's hard to do in California; it's hard to do anywhere.

During this time, I'm smoking a lot of grass. When I was first turned on to it, I couldn't believe that life could be this way. It was the most electrifying experience. It was so freeing. So what did I do for the next seven years? I smoked every day. That's typical of my personality; I'm a very addictive person. I'm surprised that I didn't do anything to kill myself. It was absolutely wonderful and when I played the piano, I could play anything I wanted to and feel good about it. It was a very healing experience; it really opened me up in a lot of ways. Unfortunately, like all those kinds of things, I abused it. If I had done it for a couple of months, or even a couple of years, it might have been OK, but I pursued it endlessly and really abused it.

I was depressed and not able to get out there and sell. It got impossible for me to go to another door, knock on it, say hello, and start talking. I just couldn't do it. So I wasn't making any money. I lost my car—repossessed. I lost my piano and some other musical equipment—repossessed.

Everything was going downhill. I wasn't making music. I was

extremely lonely, and I had a difficult time making any friends. I stayed to myself all the time.

I was coughing a lot and feeling lousy. I felt like I had tuberculosis, my lungs weren't right, I would cough up blood. I started thinking about death and just couldn't get it out of my mind. I was scared. It was the downest time in my life. Nothing worked. I felt so miserable. I decided to go home.

At home, I saw a doctor and went through a month of tests. The tests were painful, unbelievably so.

I was in my hospital room. They had opened me up to see if they could find anything. My mother was in the room when the doctor came in. He told me that they had removed part of my lung. He went over those details and told me that I probably should have some radiation. Then he gave me the prognosis: He said that I had five years to live.

I was really struggling to hold back the tears. I felt tremendous sorrow for myself and wanted to know why. How could this be? There were many, many feelings. I started to cry, and I remember feeling very ashamed that I was crying.

Once the doctor left, my parents told me they had met with him earlier. The doctor had said to them that I only had six months.

When the doctors first told me that I was going to die, I accepted it. I did my share of crying. I went through the "Why me?" and "Oh God, how can this be?" stage.

I recovered from the initial depression rather quickly. Even though the illness was just beginning, the summer was magical for me. I was by myself mostly; it was very quiet. I meditated a lot. I just sat and listened. I like listening to sounds. I was at my mother's and stepfather's house; it's a beautiful house. The countryside was great; the trees, the grass, were green and lush. The flowers were beautiful.

Soon after I got there, I had an amazing meditational experience. I had only been meditating a couple of months. It was late in the evening; my parents were asleep, and I was up and not tired. I decided to do a meditation before going to bed. Within two or three minutes, I had an incredible bodily sensation—intense joy. I'd never experienced that in my life and it lasted maybe a second, but it seemed longer. I felt so great, and it was so intense, almost sexually intense, it was amazing. Perhaps that is when the healing happened.

But I am skeptical about "single moment healings," I mean those instances of insight that you think are going to change you forever; they don't really. Over the long run, I suppose they do pile up. By the time you're ninety, you reap the benefits of them.

During this summer, I received a lot of support from my family, from my mother and stepfather and cousins. I have a strange family, but when I needed them they were there. I got a lot of goodies from being sick. It was the first time I remember getting support from them. There was a pool at the house, and my cousins would come every day and we'd go swimming.

About this time, the holistic physician I was working with made a recording for me. It did incredible things for me. It dealt with love and forgiveness, and the music hit me very, very emotionally, which isn't too hard to do. I started crying, and I was crying and crying for about a month. I was so sensitive in that month; I just cried at anything.

About a week after he gave me the tape, I was feeling very cold one night and shivering—really shivering, feeling cold or nervous. I just couldn't get warm enough.

Finally I woke my parents up. My stepfather, who I didn't always have the best relationship with, nor he with me, came out in his underwear. He sat by my bed, never said a word, and put his arm around me, and I started crying. I kept crying and crying. I cried for a total of three hours straight. My mother, of course, was really upset. She was sitting on the other side of the bed. I don't think she really understood what was going on or how to deal with it, but Roy knew. He was doing something I never expected him to do. He was a very gruff person. He has a lot of emotions, but he doesn't show them. He just sat there and never said a word, kept his arm there, and then I started to get warm, then everything was all right. He was there when I needed him. It was a great healing thing for me, for both of us. After that, we weren't the same. We were much closer, much more willing to give to each other.

It's those kinds of experiences that really heal me, those emotional, get-out-all-the-crap experiences. Since I was a young kid, I've bottled everything up, and I mean cancer is really the body destroying itself. That's exactly what you do by leaving all that shit in; you gotta get it out.

But I continued crying, like I said, for about a month, every day at the slightest thing. I never thought I had so many tears. I mean, you know, "Cry Me a River."

I was reading a lot. A friend loaned me *Seth Speaks.* It completely turned me around. I began to think that, in some way, I'm responsible for my health. I never used to think like that. In examining myself, I began to understand what part I had to play in it.

I began to look at the sources of the cancer. There were certain things my father and I had in common emotionally that weren't very good for either of us. He also died of the same kind of cancer I got. I know it sounds childish, but the cancer may have been a way of saying, "Daddy, I've caught an illness just like you did. So maybe now you'll love me." You know that New Age kind of thinking. I don't know if it's true, but it's a possibility.

Well, anyway, during this time, after my upper lobe was removed, I was getting radiation. The cancer in the lung seemed OK. After this initial round of radiation treatments, the doctors decided to give me chemotherapy. I couldn't even pronounce the damn drug. Methotrexate is now used by everybody, but at the time it was experimental. The little I knew about it frightened me. I was told that it could cause liver disorders, kidney disorders, et cetera, et cetera. When I was lying there having that stuff sucked into me, I was scared. I said to the doctor, "I don't want liver or kidney disorders. I just can't do it anymore." So I took one course of it for twenty-four hours and refused to have any more. It was my decision to make; for the first time ever, I took responsibility for my health.

When all of this started, I was very naive medically. I mean I don't think I'd been to a doctor before. So I didn't really understand how the medical establishment works. After three years, I learned.

I found a very simple thing. It sounds strange, but it's simple: Doctors are human. You invest them with so much power and magic, you put yourself in their hands, and you know they're going to cure you. When they don't, you have to decide how much of your power you want to give them.

I was at the VA hospital. It's a teaching hospital, which means these young doctors are there right out of medical school to get experience, constantly coming and going every three months. There's no opportunity to say, "Tell me what you think." You can't get a bead on someone.

The connection with medical people was not emotionally healing. There are just too many patients around. I mean, God, the hospitals are overloaded. It's just the way the system goes. The doctors figure they have to protect themselves, "You can't care too much. You can't give of yourself too much."

The cancer spread to my brain, which is a common place for lung cancer to spread in men, if they live long enough. They decided to go with the radiation, a rather heavy dosage. The thinking was: Well, he's not expected to survive anyway, and he took it well before, so give him a good dose.

When the cancer went to my eye about a year later, I said, "This is ridiculous. This is not going to be my life, once a year getting cancer. Enough of this crap."

In examining the universe, I found that things made sense; there was an order, a certain degree of stability. So when I had cancer and heard how bad it was, it just didn't make sense to me that I would have suffered all through my life and then just die. What's the point of it? It doesn't make any sense at all. So I said, "That's ridiculous, I'm not going to have that! I'm going to be well!"

I was seriously thinking of going to Mexico for Laetril. A friend had given me some tapes on relaxing and visualization from the Simontons. I had decisions to make. For some reason or other, I chose the Simontons. That was the best decision I made.

I took the Amtrak out to Fort Worth. It was a wonderful trip. I met a couple of guys, and we became fast friends. They were going to Vegas to do some gambling. It was so great. We gabbed and played cards the whole time. It was great fun. I realize now that we were all going gambling—the stakes were just different for me.

The Simontons were wonderful to me. The situation was very loving; they gave me a tremendous amount of support. Relating to people used to be one of my biggest problems—probably still is. Literally, I was scared to death of people and the world. So I stayed by myself all the time. I was lonely.

I did an awful lot of work in Texas. Group therapy was a requirement of the program. I could say what I wanted to, probably for the first time in my life. I was nervous doing it, but at least I would do it. I used to think that I was simply strange, but I discovered that there were other people who felt the same way I did. I also learned that I wasn't completely an idiot or an asshole. I feel much better about myself now, much stronger.

One of the patients there, a man in his late forties, early fifties, described a very difficult time with his mother. I had a sense that he wouldn't make it. He just couldn't get rid of his hate and anger. It was interesting to me because I had so many negative feelings for my mother. It helped me to make peace with her. She has gone her way, I mine. She doesn't understand me, I don't understand her, but that's OK. I saw that she had her own problems; the way she acted toward me wasn't anything personal—she had not wanted to deliberately hurt me. She couldn't do any better.

I learned imaging at the Simontons. I used black and white dots, not very imaginative, not very colorful. But that's what I used. I visualized my eye, 'cause at the time that's where the problem was. I could see a lot of black dots, which were the cancer cells, and they were surrounded by the white dots, which were the immune cells, and I saw them scooping up, enveloping the cancer cells, killing them and then draining them out of the body in the bloodstream. It's a very natural process, very simple.

I also learned something interesting about other cancer patients. The one common trait seems to be that they're not doing what they should be doing. They may be doing things for money, for other people, but not what they really want to do. I think people get well because they finally begin to do what they should be doing—not what other people think they should be doing, not what Mommy or Daddy want them to do.

But if you don't feel that great about yourself, about life, then you just keep putting "it" off, whatever "it" is that you really want to be doing.

I used to feel lazy about my work; I had a tremendous amount of ennui. I didn't have the same work ethic that my stepfather had, and he used to hate me for that. It's a shame he never knew that when I'm working on music or my artwork I can work all day very intensely. Because I love it, I put my heart and soul into it. It's a tremendous source of pride.

Punching a time clock or selling encyclopedias is a dead life for me. Other people can do it, it's fine, but for me it's deadly.

The Simonton program was a tremendous experiment for me. It was really the turning point. But in retrospect, I think belief has everything to do with healing. If you do a year of macrobiotics, or if you eat wheat grass, or do the Simontons, for all intents and purposes they're very similar. All that's required is your belief that it's going to work, and it'll work. You can go down to the Simontons, not believe in it, and it won't do you any good. If you come back and do macrobiotics faithfully, all of a sudden, you may be healed.

Thank God for the cancer. If it weren't for the illness, I'd probably be dead now. I was so closed down, it was a tremendous lesson. In a lot of ways, I feel very fortunate that it happened to me.

I guess it woke me up. It made me see how vulnerable I am as a human being—how vulnerable we all are.

Feeling that vulnerable is a motivating factor because there are certain things that I want to accomplish, and, if I die tomorrow, I'm not going to be able to accomplish them.

Throughout my younger life, I used to think that I had a tremendous amount of time left. Maybe I do and maybe I don't. No one ever knows that. I think it's good for me to act like I don't. You have the next minute, what else do you really have?

During the next five years, I listened to the recording of our original interview many times and felt that I got to know Joe a lot better. In reality, we had no contact during these years. When I called Joe to ask if we could arrange another interview, I had hoped we could do it over the phone. He was nearly 500 miles away, and I believed then that I understood the essence of his story. Joe let me know that he would be glad to speak with me again, in person. He didn't like the phone. He invited me to his apartment.

Joe's neighborhood was made up of working-class people and graduate students. He lived on the top floor of a triplex. Joe had told me to yell up for him when I got there; the doorbell wasn't working. When I arrived, however, he was waiting at the door.

The apartment was modest, too sparse to seem disheveled. Walking into his living room, by way of the bedroom, there was a presence that couldn't have been more surprising than seeing an elephant. The brownstone was dilapidated, the stairway to the third floor narrow and windy, and the living room tiny. But the piano was a baby grand. Joe laughed when he saw my reaction. He explained how he had hired a seventy-foot crane and taken out windows, casings and all, to move his old friend in.

Before the recorder was turned on, Joe had something to tell me. He had quit smoking a few years ago. He had taken advantage of the three-week head start given to him by a bad case of bronchitis and sore throat. He finished this story by saying, "Thank God for the bronchitis."

His home was filled with his musical instruments and paintings. We went into the kitchen, where we talked around a kitchen table stacked with charcoal drawings. The conversation was easy. We had a certain history together now.

After some internal struggle, I put my interview format aside to focus on Joe's music and art. Once in his living space, I could understand, in a way that had not been possible before, the significance of aesthetics in his life. If I really wanted to know who Joe was and why he believed he recovered, I had best listen to what Joe had to say about creativity.

Joe began again by telling me about his everyday life.

I really love getting up in the morning and practicing. I just love it. In the evening, I do my artwork. During the afternoon, I do some teaching and practice when I can.

Since I last saw you, I've practiced every day of my life except vacations. And on vacations, if I can, I practice. I've been doing that for the past eight years. It will be part of my life for the rest of my life.

The healing opened me up to my emotions, and it comes out in my music. Or maybe I was healed because I opened up. What did I tell you last time? [Joe laughed.] I certainly have intense feelings, and they get expressed through my music and my artwork—more so all the time.

I have a new piano teacher. My first teacher was a technocrat. He taught me all the things to do and not to do; it was necessary that I have that.

In the sixth year, I started studying with this fellow who uses his own feelings to teach. So now I'm much more willing to express my feelings at the instrument than before. It's difficult for me to do, but it's coming. I have been called gifted. But we all have this gift, it's just a matter of finding your own form.

After I've really, really expressed myself, I'm always embarrassed. Very. I feel I've exposed myself to other people. I can't stand to be there; I'd rather get out of the room.

If I've put my ego into it, I'll stay to accept the applause and all that crap. And if I've played with any kind of emotion, if I've done my best to feel, I'm very embarrassed. But that's also when music is beautiful.

Nothing's more scary, but, on the other hand, the rewards are unmatched. There's nothing better in the world than playing like that—nothing. That is the whole point of it.

At those moments, I'm seeing myself revealed to myself for the first time. It makes me think of a concert I went to with Keith Jarrett at Symphony Hall. He played an encore piece that reduced me to tears. I never heard anything so beautiful, so sensitive, so alive. It was an absolutely incredible experience. Whether he felt that way or not, I don't know, and it doesn't really matter. But I assume he did. You can't receive that kind of communication without someone else sending it.

That's the highest and the best communication possible. It's very hard to achieve and not every piece was like that. I don't think it could have been.

That's a beautiful work, that's communication. It is what being human is about.

Since my illness, I have gotten much closer to my natural human self. Your natural self has a lot of creativity, a lot of intelligence, a lot of emotionality, a lot of spirituality. We all have this innate wisdom, but over the years it becomes encrusted with so much crap that we lose access. When you rediscover this inner self, you suddenly can do things that were impossible before. It happens naturally. The more you love yourself, the more you can get in touch with who you basically are.

If I had died from the cancer, it would have been a shame because I have learned so much since the illness. I would have missed the opportunity to discover a little bit about who I am. As far as I'm concerned, I'd be happy if I never died. But I feel better knowing that I have done something to find out what life is all about.

I move slow, and I move cautiously, but I'm moving.

OBSERVATIONS

Joe believes that cancer is the body eating itself up. To survive, he was clear: He had to "get the shit out." He needed to find an outlet for his toxic feelings, and he needed to feel better about himself. The urgency of the situation freed him and also compelled him to begin the metamorphosis he felt was necessary for continued life.

Music was Joe's primary way to communicate his innermost feelings and release what was inside. Creative expression was a vehicle he could use to expel the feelings that ate at him; and it was the means to connect with the world. In the past, he had always wanted to make music, but somehow he would sabotage any sustained effort. Giving free reign to this life force also meant that he was no longer at war with himself. Energy that he previously expended in his ongoing battle with himself could be focused toward healing.

Joe also began a struggle to communicate more openly with others. The poignancy of the moment he was given the diagnosis suggests just how repressed he was then. Despite the devastation of the news, he attempted to hold back his feelings and felt ashamed of himself for crying. Joe is still not satisfied with his level of interpersonal functioning, but he relates very differently now. Indeed his willingness to expose how closed he used to be demonstrates how much he now desires to share more of himself.

Most of all, Joe has changed the way he feels about himself. To use his own metaphor, Joe's insides were no longer filled with shit once he realized that he wasn't a complete asshole. He knows he has work to do in the area of self-esteem, but he is in process. He attempts to overcome his destructive gut feelings of inadequacy with his more intellectual understanding that he is a valuable human being. Through meditation, he practices being with himself without judgment or attachment.

Before the cancer, Joe had little reason to live. He was depressed, had no meaningful relationships, no work, and no purpose. It seemed that life could not possibly get worse—until he found out he had terminal cancer. Finally he had nothing more to be afraid of; there was nothing left to lose. Living without fear, he experienced a strange new sense of freedom. So, while most of us could imagine feeling only horror during the days after a life-threatening diagnosis, Joe's summer was filled with peace and magic.

Extraordinary healing, and perhaps all healing is a creative act.

Sickness is transformed into health, a new state of being is created. According to Pablo Picasso, "Every act of creation is first of all an act of destruction." Before Joe could create his new self, the old self had to be destroyed or at least pronounced terminal. He thanked God for the cancer because it let him know that he was leading a dead life and that his body would survive only if he changed.

Research cannot yet evaluate the healing power of creativity, but anecdotal accounts are impressive. In one such account, Norman Cousins visited with the aged Pablo Casals, who suffered arthritis that swelled his fingers and clenched his fists. Yet these infirmities were transcended when he made music. Cousins wrote:

> He stretched his arms in front of him and extended his fingers. Then the spine straightened and he stood up and went to his cello.
>
> He began to play. His fingers, hands, and arms were in sublime coordination as they responded to the demands of his brain for the controlled beauty of movement and tone. Any cellist thirty years his junior would have been proud to have such extraordinary physical command.
>
> Twice in one day I had seen the miracle. A man almost ninety, beset with the infirmities of old age, was able to cast off his afflictions, at least temporarily, because he knew he had something of overriding importance to do. There was no mystery about the way it worked, for it happened every day. Creativity for Pablo Casals was the source of his own cortisone. It is doubtful whether any antiinflammatory medication he would have taken would have been as powerful or as safe as the substances produced by the interaction of his mind and body. . . . He was caught up in his own creativity, in his own desire to accomplish a specific purpose, and the effect was both genuine and observable.

The task in music, in healing, in life, is to discover a truth that resonates to one's very core. The creative process informs us that the truth is all around us. Joe's understanding of improvisational jazz told him that there was no right way to play a melody, no single reality, and no single way to fight a disease. Roger von Oech, author of *A Whack on the Side of the Head*, tells a Sufi story that is apropos:

Two men had an argument. To settle the matter, they went to a Sufi judge for arbitration. The plaintiff made his case. He was very eloquent and persuasive in his reasoning. When he finished, the judge nodded in approval and said, "That's right, that's right."

On hearing this, the defendant jumped up and said, "Wait a second, judge, you haven't even heard my side of the case yet." So the judge told the defendant to state his case. And he, too, was very persuasive and eloquent. When he finished, the judge said, "That's right, that's right."

When the clerk of court heard this, he jumped up and said, "Judge, they both can't be right." The judge looked at the clerk of court and said, "That's right, that's right."

Joe didn't reduce his choice to "scientific" medicine vs. "holistic" approaches. To divine a right answer for himself, Joe probed within, conducted a personal assessment, then concluded what treatment was necessary. Thus chemotherapy didn't seem right but radiation did. His diet wasn't an important focus of concern, but visualization and meditation were.

He unequivocally asserted that the source of his cancer was emotional rather than environmental. In light of the fact that there was no concrete data to support this claim, his resoluteness as well as his ability to act in accordance with this belief was remarkable. His strength is all the bolder when contrasted with how unempowered he felt before the illness. One example: Prior to the cancer, he was not even able to maintain possession of his musical instruments, the symbol and tool of his creativity. Once he became gravely ill, however, a time when the most confident of people doubt their ability to make a difference, Joe declared with absolute authority that he was going to be well.

Whether one can really know with 100 percent accuracy the origin of an illness as complex as cancer remains a mystery. But, as Joe suggests, the "truth" of his belief system may have been less important than the strength of his convictions. His beliefs may have created their own reality, a reality that served him well.

One final note concerning Joe's strong beliefs and his decision to discontinue chemotherapy soon after he began: It would be a mistake to generalize from his experience. He decided that he needed to stop, but he would not advise someone else to do the same thing. In fact, Joe later decided that especially heavy doses of radiation were in his best interest. Gregory A. Curtis, M.D., deputy director of the National Cancer Institute's Division of Cancer Treatment, offers some compelling reasons to continue with recommended treatment: "During the 1950s, surgery and radiotherapy cured approximately 30 percent of cancer patients. Over the past thirty years, the improvements in radiotherapy, and the important discovery that drugs (chemotherapy) could actually cure advanced cancer have improved the curability rate to 50 percent."*

Nearly 2,000 years ago, the Greek physician, Galen, postulated that depressed or melancholic women were more likely to develop breast cancer. Since then, many researchers and practitioners have suggested a relationship between cancer and personality types. Although there is considerable agreement on these personal characteristics, there is still no consensus in the medical community as to whether certain emotions predispose one to cancer or influence recovery.

Associating personality styles with the development of cancer or any other illness is an area that needs to be approached cautiously; it is ripe with the potential for abuse. Blaming the sick for their condition (or causing the sick to blame themselves) is a most destructive distortion of the concept.

The fact that emotional characteristics may be associated with cancer development for some people does not necessarily have any implications for the individual with cancer. In my own work with cancer patients, I have met many people who do not possess any of the characteristics of the "typical" cancer patient. Notwithstanding these comments, it would be shortsighted to omit a discussion of these personality variables, for the generalities presented may offer some personal insight to the healthy as well as the sick.

In years of work with cancer patients, Lawrence LeShan developed a comprehensive cancer personality profile. In one project, he and a colleague studied 250 cancer patients. They found that the following

---

*Dr. Curtis's comment does not contradict the fact that we are failing to make any real progress in the battle with cancer. Consider that in the United States in 1983 there were 855,000 new cancer cases and 440,000 people died from the disease. By 1988, with steady increases every year, there were 985,000 new cases and 494,000 deaths. The gains in treatment have not kept pace with the increases in the number of new cases.

pattern existed with 62 percent of the cancer patients compared with only 10 percent of the control group. Joe's history conforms almost perfectly with their findings:

There has been significant trauma by the age of seven that disrupts the formation of basic trust. Development of self-hatred.

Joe's parents separate. He is separated from his brother as well, and sent to parochial school, where he is abused. Joe assumes he deserves the treatment he receives.

Relationships with mother and/or father are distant and hostile. The individual learns that intimate personal relationships are not possible.

He sees his mother rarely and his father practically not at all. He has no one with whom he can really relate.

As a young adult, the establishment of a singularly important object relationship (a profession, a person, a project). Great emotional dependence on this relationship.

His music becomes the central focus of his life.

Loss of this relationship, accompanied by very severe depression.

Joe stops making music. His instruments are repossessed. He sees no way out.

In addition to these characteristics, many cancer professionals believe that cancer patients consistently suppress their emotions, especially feelings of anger. In his research with 500 cancer patients, LeShan maintains that they all shared a common characteristic—an inadequate outlet for emotional expression.

Since at least 100 different kinds of cancer have been identified, a question arises: Do the emotional characteristics of the person with lung cancer seem to conform to the personality profile of other cancer patients? Dr. David Kissen focused his research exclusively on the psychology of lung cancer patients. He found that they, too, were emotionally constricted and had great difficulty expressing their emotions.

Whether the qualities cited predispose one to cancer or influence recovery is not known. In trying to understand Joe's process, however, it is apparent that the qualities he changed in fighting his disease are also the ones usually attributed to the cancer personality. Most significantly, Joe found a meaningful way to express himself. Intimate human

expression usually takes place between two people, but Joe's relationship with music seemed to fulfill his need. A test of intimacy in any
relationship is: Do we dare show our vulnerability? Does the relationship provide a means to make our real selves known? Not only can Joe
reveal his known self through his music, he makes contact with previous
undiscovered facets of himself: "I'm seeing myself revealed to myself
for the first time." Joe may not connect intimately with another human
being, but his music encourages him to find his own truth. And, as Joe
tells us, that's what being human is about.

Joe reached out and received some important help along the way. At a
time when he was most committed to recovery, but also most ill, he
attended the Simonton Cancer Center, now located in the Pacific
Palisades, California. Back then, it was one of the few well-credentialed,
holistically oriented cancer centers.

The thrust of the treatment (clearly outlined in the Simontons' book
Getting Well Again) is to help the patient acquire a different self-image
and gain confidence that recovery is possible. Expressing feelings is
considered essential. The Simonton approach incorporates counseling,
meditation, imaging, diet, and exercise. They also recommend that their
patients take time to play.

The Simontons conducted a study of 159 "terminally ill" patients
who received treatment at their clinic. At the time they reported their
results, sixty-three were alive, with an average survival time of 24.4
months. The ninety-six patients who died had an average longevity of
20.3 months. If these same patients had been treated with only standard
medical procedures, their anticipated survival time would have been
twelve months. Perhaps most outstanding is that for the patients still
alive, 51 percent had resumed the same level of activity that they
enjoyed prior to their diagnosis.

Since the program attempts to actualize theories about the power of
the mind to heal, it is not surprising that their approach has received
harsh criticism. Refuting the validity of the Simontons' research, some
critics charge that their patients are more motivated and probably in
better health than the average "terminal" patient. Since their patients
come from all over the United States, indeed from all over the world,
they are obviously well enough to make the journey. The critics are
presumably impugning the motives of the caregivers when they contend
that their program is exorbitantly expensive. At $3250.00 for five and a

half days for two (the patient must be accompanied by a support person), the program is very expensive, but so are most forms of treatment. For example, Harvard-affiliated McLean Hospital charges $18,000 for a five-week inpatient psychiatric program, a daily rate that is comparable to the Simonton program. And the expense of either is only about half the daily cost of a room in intensive care at many major hospitals.

The Simontons provided a loving atmosphere while they encouraged Joe to pursue his deepest desires. To stay alive and thrive, one needs to have a reason to live. Rollo May, an existential psychologist who himself recovered from a life-threatening illness, believes that the patient who is deeply involved with someone or something will experience the best outcome. May says that passionate caring, such as the feeling Joe has for his music, "fights against death, fights always to assert its own vitality, accepts no 'three-score and ten' or other timetable on life." Joe wishes to live, in part, so that he can continue to make music. Caring may be the force that catalyzes the will to live.

There is wisdom in listening to one's heart. The problem is how to tune in, especially when it concerns a choice of life work. Many people don't know what they really want to do. Those who come in touch with their true desire may find that it won't happen without a frightening leap of faith. The quest is well worth the effort, for anything less will cause discontent. As Abraham Maslow, the father of self-actualization theory, tells us, "A musician must make music, an artist must paint, a poet must write if he is to be ultimately at peace with himself. What a man can be, he must be."

RELATED RESEARCH

Various studies suggest that there is a relationship between cancer and emotions. Three long-term studies are particularly evocative:

The original focus of a Johns Hopkins Medical School research project begun in 1946 was heart disease. Dr. Caroline Thomas postulated that since certain physical conditions (such as high blood pressure) could forecast future heart problems, perhaps emotional factors were also predictive. To test this hypothesis, she conducted personality assessments of 1337 students graduating from medical school between 1948 and 1964. When she began analyzing the results in the mid-seventies, more than 25 years since she started tracking the subjects, the results were both unexpected and significant. Most outstanding were the emotional commonalities of the students who developed cancer. She discovered that they seldom demonstrated strong emotions. Their lack of familial closeness—especially their remoteness from parents—was also striking.

Another long-term study was undertaken by researchers (Richard Shekelle and others) from the University of Chicago, Yale Medical School, and Harvard Medical School. Beginning in 1957, psychological tests were administered to 2,020 men. Their physical health histories were tracked for the next seventeen years. The researchers found that men who showed signs of clinical depression were twice as likely to die from cancer. This was true even after the statistics had been adjusted for age, cigarette smoking, alcohol use, occupation, and familiar cancer history.

For five years researchers H. Steven Greer and Tina Morris followed breast cancer patients at Kings College Hospital in London. Individuals who did the worst had given up or were stoic (which is essentially a stance of not expressing emotions). Patients who did the best maintained a determined attitude and generally believed that they could beat the disease.

LINDSEY REYNOLDS

For the next five years I lived the vast majority of time as though my insides were being eaten by foxes. That's how sharp and persistent the pain was. There was nothing sophisticated, rebellious, or superficial about it. It was just agonizing.

Lindsey Reynolds

The diagnostic consensus among psychiatrists who treated Lindsey Reynolds was schizophrenia.* But in the world of mental health, diagnosis is more art than science. When a case is difficult to evaluate, and Lindsey Reynolds's case was very difficult, clinicians will frequently defer their own opinion to that of whoever conducted the last assessment rather than risk conflict. There is another reason to question her schizophrenia label. Twenty-five years ago, the last time Lindsey was in a mental hospital, schizophrenia was (and sometimes still is) a catchall category used when a more precise diagnosis eluded the clinician.

Lindsey is now a mental health professional herself. She believes that borderline personality disorder** more accurately describes her former condition. After reading more than two hundred pages of her medical records and meeting with her former psychotherapist, I concur with her opinion.

*Schizophrenia is characterized by the withdrawal from consensually validated reality. It involves bizarre delusions, auditory hallucinations, and/or incoherence with affect that is flat or inappropriate.

**Borderline personality disorder may be evidenced by behavior that is physically harmful to oneself, such as suicidal gestures or self-mutilation. There can be strong mood shifts fluctuating from normal mood to depression, anger, or anxiety. Relationships are generally unstable, and anger may be intense and out of control.

93

Since the professionals who are familiar with the case do not dispute
its essence, pinpointing the diagnosis is really not necessary. For there is
unanimity of opinion: Lindsey suffered from severe mental illness, and
the prognosis was very bleak.

I asked three highly skilled colleagues, all psychotherapists, to review
the case material. Lindsey's outcome was remarkable, they agreed. I
asked the therapists to look to their own professional experiences for
comparisons. None of them had ever worked with a patient who made
such an extraordinary recovery. Her history actually serves to inform us
all that emotional health is possible even for those who are struggling
with the most serious forms of mental illness.

I spent a great deal of time with Lindsey and her family—more than
150 hours. Her twenty-three-year marriage to Stephen has survived not
just her illness but her health as well. I met with members of her
community, both professional and personal. My assessment of her
present level of functioning, then, is based on an enormous quantity of
data.

Karl Menninger speaks about people who are "weller than well."
These are individuals who have recovered from a serious illness and
now demonstrate new strength and vigor. We have each experienced this
phenomenon at a personal level. If we gash ourselves, a scar develops
as the final stage of healing. This new skin is stronger than the original.
When we have the chicken pox, measles, or various other infectious
illnesses, our bodies grow stronger and more resistant through the
healing process; we will never again be subjected to that particular
disease. Menninger might have suggested that Lindsey is emotionally
"weller than well." People who know her intimately refer to her as a
"wise woman."

Lindsey is the executive director of a small mental health center.
Although administrative tasks demand much of her time, she supervises
other psychotherapists and continues to work with a limited number of
patients herself. A local therapist communicated ultimate faith in Lindsey's
competence as both a professional and a human being. He shared with
me, "If I ever felt that I was going over the edge into madness, Lindsey
is the one person I would want to be there."

The quality that I found most attractive and perhaps most difficult to
capture on paper was her relentless pursuit to make sense of the past.
She does not merely tell her story. She processes events as she talks,

making new connections, drawing conclusions, and discovering new insight into who she is. She applies this same life force to understanding others, without judgment or evaluation.

Lindsey is tall, about five feet eight, with classically attractive features. High cheek bones draw one into her dark brown eyes. Her face is calm and ageless, without a hint of her past except for a hairline scar that runs from the top of one eyebrow across her entire forehead.

Lindsey began by talking about her family:

Part of my confusion in growing up was that my childhood always *looked* good—to me and to everybody else. The issues in the family were subtle ones. My parents were nice people. There was no serious abuse, but they were not really present to protect or nurture their children. They were very engaged in being the young beautiful couple with children who should please others.

There were always maids in my house so I was not without nurturance. They were the ones who took care of my bumps and scratches, and they were the ones who fed me dinner when we weren't being served in the big dining room. My attachment to these women was very intense, but these women would leave; they would be fired or just move on.

Alcohol was always flowing. Alcohol was the mode of relating between my parents, among their friends. They would get drunk and lose their inhibitions. My father might make a seductive remark, say something about how nice my legs were or point them out to his friends. It was far from incest, but I never had the feeling that the line was very clear. When I was about ten, my family's lawyer, a man named Harry, would sexually molest me: grab me, kiss me, touch me, nothing much worse than that, but it was terrifying.

About five years ago, I told my mother about Harry. Her response, her entire response, was, "Doesn't surprise me. Harry was after me all the time." There was no surprise, no horror, no question, no awareness that mothers protect their children in these ways.

I think there was an incest culture in my family. I learned that my brother had attempted intercourse with my sister. This does not happen in a family where there are clear sexual boundaries. As an adult, my brother explained to me that he had not been attracted to me because I was overweight. He said it as if he didn't want to hurt my feelings. He implied that otherwise this would have happened between us as well.

I was not a happy kid. Trouble was evident by the time I was five or six. I stole food from stores, from school, from friends' houses. I got caught many times, but my mother sloughed it off. She'd get mad but then say it was just normal stuff that kids do—which it wasn't. I think it served my mother and father not to understand me. They did not have to do anything as long as they did not understand me.

I was not a popular kid. Since I was fat, I assume I must have been eating constantly. I'd go to the dentist and have as many as thirty cavities. Later on, I questioned whether I was really trying to make it impossible for me to eat. I remember times when, because of my weight, kids would throw stones at me. It was very cruel.

The only times I remember as happy were when I was swimming at our country club. I was a very good swimmer, and my parents and their friends gave me a lot of recognition for that. I developed intense fantasies that we would move close to the country club. After school one day, my parents told me that we were moving there. I think that really set me up to believe that I could cause things by merely believing them. I also decided that we were moving because my parents were ashamed of me and we needed to get out of town because of my criminal proclivities.

We moved when I was ten years old. I remember a cousin who was very beautiful and popular. I watched her often, and I thought, well, I'm going to be like her. I made a very conscious decision to change my personality—to be outgoing, to use my sense of humor, to become popular at the new school. I loved it there. I was well liked, both by teachers and by kids. We had a huge country home. I could walk to the country club. I was very happy; life was going well.

It also meant that my mother and father had really entered the fast lane financially as well as socially. My brother tells me that there was a party a week at our house. Famous people came. There was always a lot of alcohol. It was very intense.

The circumstances around my father's death were all so agonizing. It was a terrible loss.

I was starting my sophomore year at this private school, when my teacher, an English woman, announced that a girl coming to our class had been in a plane crash. She was sitting next to her mother, and her mother was killed. The teacher wanted us all to be extremely giving and kind to this girl. I was blown away by the incredible drama of this story, more than by any real empathy for this girl, although there were probably moments of that, too. I wanted a drama of that magnitude. So I began to fantasize such a drama.

The loss for me that would be as devastating, as I thought of it, would be the loss of my father. So I began to have active fantasies of his death. When he died, I felt certain that I was the cause. I had killed him.

He was vacationing in the islands with my mother. They were dancing at a party when he said he was tired. He went up to bed. When she went up an hour later, he was dead.

Since my mother was not home, she called a good friend to pick me up from school and tell me what had happened. Instead, her friend called me on the phone, told me my father was dead, then left me at school for hours before coming to collect me.

It was raining, cold, and raw on the day of his funeral. At the church, I asked my mother if I could cry since we were in public. She said yes, but I think the question indicates the inhibition in the family.

A lot of people went to the grave, to the burial. After his body was lowered, everyone paired up and walked away together. I was left there alone. No one came to me. The minister, who I was not particularly fond of, saw me standing alone and did not come over. I was paralyzed. So this oversight, which is all it was, added to the belief that I had killed my father. On some level, I believed that these people knew it, so they left me there to be alone.

The belief that I had killed my father became an increasingly entrenched secret until I was exploding with madness.

Our whole financial picture, which had been pretty rosy, was no longer so. There was no life insurance; my mother had to go to work. Everything had to change.

I remember an extremely humiliating moment when I went back to school. Every month we would be weighed in the gymnasium. You had to stand in line, and it felt like a very public thing. After I stepped on the scale, the gym teacher said, "Oh good, you haven't lost any weight." I took that to mean that if I had really cared about my father, as opposed to being a murderess, I would have lost weight. In fact, because of this terrific anxiety I was eating all the time and actually gained weight.

Nobody except a few friends knew that I was in trouble. In my junior year, I went into a massive rebellion, skipped school constantly, and nearly got expelled. But the following year, as a senior, despite my emotional turmoil my grades improved. And the comments from the teachers were positive.

My grades improved because the previous summer I worked at a Howard Johnson's on the Thruway, with ice cream up to my elbows and no air conditioning. I decided if I didn't do something about school, I wouldn't get into a good college and it would be my fate to work forever at Howard Johnson's, which was my definition of hell.

All the outward indicators belied what was going on internally. My physical appearance changed drastically. I went to my father's doctor. Those weight reduction quacks were very popular then. He put me on Dexadrine, speed. I lost forty pounds. I was wearing a size 18 when I began my senior year, and I graduated in a size 10 dress. Suddenly I was being rushed by men. There had been no gradual introduction to this world, so I did not know what was going on.

When I got to Bryn Mawr, I was struggling with the deep agonies and confusion about who I was, questioning why I felt so apart from others.

I sought out and spent a great deal of time with a very wealthy family. At some level, I'm sure the attempt was to regain my privileged status. The wife was as good as could be. She was extremely kind and she really did love me.

She had no idea what was going on. Her husband was sexually exploiting me, and I did not know what to do. It made me crazy. He introduced me to fellatio. I was terrified and repelled; I felt myself to be an adultress and I thought of myself as special. Despite the terror, there was too much drawing me there, in terms of security, to stay away. In some ways, I know now that all of my childhood was a preparation for this. It got pretty scuzzy. I stopped going there when he began making passes at my friends. It turns out that this guy eventually went to jail for sexually assaulting young children.

I met a very good-looking boy from Tufts. My first experience of sexual intercourse was with this boy—in essence a date rape. We had fucked that night, and the next morning I tried to make myself believe that I was in love with him. But he was extremely rejecting and pushed me away.

It seems there was always external confirmation of my worst fears. I went to a class and the professor said, in relation to a story we were reading, that any woman who lets herself be seduced is a fool.

Over Christmas break, I found out that my best friend, Gloria, was not returning; she went to Austin Riggs instead. At that time, my whole image of mental hospitals was the snake pit variety. It scared the hell out of me because I knew it was inevitable for me as well. She and I used to talk about this, and we both agreed that of the two of us, I was the more disturbed.

My myths about mental hospitals were dispelled very quickly when I visited Gloria at Austin Riggs, which was just like a first-class hotel. I spent the night illegally there; they didn't know I was there. I was introduced to marijuana for the first time. I also remember seeing a woman break a Coke bottle and then cut her wrists with one of the jagged edges.

At Bryn Mawr, I took a bunch of sleeping pills. But I did it right in front of a friend. I had my stomach pumped and made up some absurd excuse for my actions. This happened many times, and it's just amazing the willingness of hospital personnel to buy the most absurd stories. I don't know what I said, but it couldn't have been too brilliant. I started breaking windows at school and I'd say that I'd had a terrible nightmare, and it happened by mistake.

I engaged a professor in this whole drama. I told him what was going on but swore him to secrecy, which he never should have agreed to. So it took a long time for this to come out. I was walking in front of cars. As I recall, I was still taking speed all of this time. Finally this professor called the psychiatrist. I was a mess, so the psychiatrist really had no choice. He threw me out.

I had been calling my mother nightly, crying on the phone, saying I need to come home, I need to come home. She would tell me to just finish my sophomore year.

After I got kicked out, I told her what the psychiatrist had said. She responded, "Oh, don't be ridiculous. You just need a rest or something." Desperate, I went over to a psychiatric clinic myself. They refused to treat me because I was under age.

Finally my mother agreed to have me see a friend of hers who was head of psychiatry at Riverview Hospital. The guy was very good to me.

He said that I was in great need of therapy, and my mother listened to that. They assigned me to see Richard Jameson for outpatient therapy. He was chief resident at Riverview. Within three weeks, I was admitted to the hospital after I cut myself with a Coke bottle.

I wouldn't speak to Jameson at all. Part of that was my increasing despair. Part of it was "come and find me." Don't make me do so much of the work, just come and find me, make some effort, which he didn't make. He made effort to the level he knew to make it, but it was meager.

I had no stake in changing. My reality was that I lived in this immense agony and that would not change, could not change. Change only meant that I wouldn't be in a hospital, that I would be at home, which meant that I would be unsafe again.

I was such an awful human being, so flawed, so to be despised I did not think of it in terms of sickness because that suggested the possibility of being well.

I did a lot of adolescent acting out, which were really the only good times. Other than injections of sedation, the acting out was my only relief. I would sneak alcohol in, or run away, or just be a pain in the ass. They would get angry and tell me that it had to stop, in a stern nonwishy-washy sort of way. So I'd have a straight-out, wished-for parental interaction. Those moments were very wonderful to me.

I was put in seclusion for most of the time I was there. That's not as stark as it sounds. There were a lot of people around. In fact, the attention was more concentrated and reliable there than anyplace else.

But there was a sexual incident there. An aide would wait until the sleeping medication had taken effect and then whatever happened, happened. There are some vague memories, but there was something sexual. Again, this was somebody that I really cared for who was doing this. Each time something new happened, it was just more confirmation that I was to blame. It never occurred to me that I wasn't. All kinds of things came together to convince me that there really was something terribly wrong with me, that I was a perverse, seducing-the-world, murdering human being. Other than that, I had no problems with my self-image.

My brother would take me out on visits for a few hours. On one visit, I bought a razor blade. I came back to the seclusion room and put it under a loose tile. A few nights later, I cut myself up pretty badly. I cut my wrists and my arms. That time it took maybe twelve to fifteen stitches. They would get so angry and be very punitive, so they would often sew me up without anesthesia.

At that point, these gestures were an attempt to extract more from the system or more from the people I really cared about. They asked me where I kept the razor blade because I was in my pajamas in a seclusion room. They couldn't understand it because there was nothing in the room except a bed. I showed them the loose tile.

One day, I sat in there and took up every other tile in the room. By the time they came in to see me, I had them stacked all around the room. They flipped out, they were so ripped. That kind of acting out always gave me some moment of peace and normalcy—gave it not to anybody else, but to me. But then it would just come back on me, because somebody that I cared about almost got fired for not watching me more closely.

They put me in a different room with only a mattress on the floor. I was stripped down to that. This was proof that I was the sickest, the most profound human being in the place. This was proof that I was suffering worse than anyone else, so in a way it was confirming. The same set of facts were also terrifying.

The only time I remember feeling really connected to Jameson, and I doubt that he knew this, was after I tore up all the tiles. He came in, and he was ripped. He gave me this incredible lecture about the way I was behaving and told me that he was having a hard time keeping me there. Apparently, he was fighting to keep them from sending me to Bellevue. I felt very connected at that moment in time. Of course, it led to more acting out, because that was exactly the kind of connection I needed.

I think they were concerned that I was untreatable. I was probably seen as privileged, spoiled, and quite sick. Hopelessness was communicated. I mean my shrink, Jameson, would come in and spend ten minutes trying to reach me. If he didn't reach me in ten minutes, and that time got shorter and shorter, he'd leave. I was passive, depressed, and withdrawn. I was angry and avoidant. If he didn't bring much energy into the relationship, I didn't have it to give. I mean he had to lend everything. He wasn't able to, or he did not understand how to do it. He began to rely on electric shock treatment.

The shock treatment was not helpful. I don't think that there was any justification for them. The therapist did not know how to treat me, and so he became desperate. My stay at Riverview was running out. They kept patients for only three months. Jameson probably feared that, without successful treatment of some sort, I was looking at a very long hospitalization someplace, which indeed turned out to be the case.

They told me that if I refused to go to Mountain Brook Hospital voluntarily, they would take court action to commit me. Commitment laws were quite lax then, and they could have committed me on the basis of two psychiatrists saying that I needed to be institutionalized, which wouldn't have been hard.

I made all kinds of threats—"You'll never get me there alive," "I'll throw myself out of the car." I had a real premium on drama. I do think that there can be confusion on the part of caregivers when they think of drama as simple attention seeking. That attachment to drama is life affirming, if you don't kill yourself in the process. It has something to do with the richness of life. It doesn't cut just one way.

My drama was of the order of getting drunk or throwing myself out of a car or cutting myself up. It involved some secondary gains, attempting to get some kind of a payoff. But my acts were also filled with an enormous amount of despair and self-hatred. I was dangerous to myself; there was no question about that.

They sedated me very heavily and folded me into the back of my mother's car with this nurse that I liked very much. They locked the doors. I was transported to Mountain Brook.

I tell you, Mountain Brook was quite a shock.

The casual observer cannot see it, but a relationship I developed with a therapist there was the cornerstone of my healing. When I tell this story, and I have told this story in the past, people think that Mountain Brook was the end of my trials because it was such a significant time. In fact, it was just the beginning.

When I got there, a rather officious-looking nurse led me to a locked ward. I think I was disappointed because she, like the other nurses, wore regular clothes. There were no uniforms to sanctify the illness. I was put into a group room under constant observation. There were some very crazy women in that group room—me among them. Since Mountain Brook was one of the few private hospitals that still had locked units, it got some of the most disturbed people.

When I first arrived, Will Goodman, the man who would be my psychiatrist, was on leave. Many patients and some of the nurses told me he was one of the best at the institution. Via the hospital grapevine, I learned that he wasn't there because his brother, the person with whom he was closest in the world, had been killed in a car accident a week earlier.

The two psychiatrists I had seen before, Jameson at Riverview and Larry Nash, who was filling in until my psychiatrist returned, both happened to be very good-looking, so I at least wanted someone with movie-star good looks. I also had come from a fairly privileged, not always wealthy, Greenwich, Connecticut, family that was very sophisticated. So I was shocked when Will Goodman walked into the interviewing room. He was plain-looking, he had thinning blond hair, glasses, and a very noticeable midwestern accent. I thought: Oh, my God, what have they done? This is never going to work, this absolute hick from wherever.

I had learned—the way you learn the lay of the landscape, you don't notice it, you don't study it, but you just learn it—I had learned in my time with psychiatrists that they really did enjoy statements of angst and lots of affective expression. There was subtle reinforcement to express yourself in these ways. It was very rare, I felt, that the communication was real. It was a communication where you performed your illness and they commented on it.

In my initial interview with him, I remember saying, "I love my mother." I repeated that many times. Finally, he said, "You told me that already." I was so startled by his realness. It was a bit sharp and impatient. Very different from the analytic principles of aloofness and distance that were so popular at the time. He unnerved me.

I think I liked him from the time he said that.

There were also normative differences between the hospitals. Riverview Hospital was a New York, Jewish, Puerto Rican, university-affiliated establishment. This was upstate New York, WASP, and I think everything was supposed to quiet down. There was very little encouragement of acting out.

Goodman took me in hand immediately. No risks would be taken, he said. If I acted out, I would go to Carlson II. There were lots of levels at Mountain Brook. I was on a unit called Carlson I; the only unit that was worse, sort of the Bellevue of Mountain Brook, was Carlson II.

The issues were my safety, my security, and who was in control. He established that very quickly. During my second interview, Goodman told me I would be there for two years. I was both alarmed and relieved. With Jameson, I was too much in control. I really had the upper hand in all the worst ways—like a spoiled child. Goodman saw that and didn't have much appreciation for the Greenwich entitlement. That was partly cultural. In New York, where Jameson lived, my kind of brattiness was commonplace. But now I had this midwesterner who didn't like it. It was not OK with him. I needed someone to be in control, someone who didn't waver. Had I felt any chink in the armor, I would have gone into a panic.

Right away, we had a few run-ins. I was on constant observation, suicide watch, which meant the nurses even came to the bathroom with me. Not only did I get constipated, I couldn't pee. I argued with him to remove me from constant surveillance.

He said, "No, you're just too big a risk. I won't do it."

I protested, "This is getting dangerous."

He said, "You'll pee. You'll adjust."

I wanted desperately to get out of the group room because of this woman who was snoring. But he wouldn't take me out of there either. The only plea he did in fact grant me was sleeping medication, partly because I had a long history of not sleeping well and partly because he knew there was this class A snorer in the room. Through our negotiations, I learned that he was very tough, but he wasn't going to be tough without reflection or without care. I very rapidly felt protected by this. For my whole life, especially after my father's death, it seemed no one was in control, no one was watching out for me.

I acted out very little. I didn't need to. He made it clear that he knew I was out of control; I didn't need to prove it to him in any way. He saw me three times a week; the norm was twice. That gave me the status of clearly being disturbed. The precautions when I came in that were so much more rigid than what other people got, his telling me that I'd be there for two years—these were ways of saying that he got the message.

I think his communication, his personality, the nature of the institution itself, the fact that I was away from my family and he had taken parental control, all lowered my anxiety to something that was much more tolerable.

I arrived in July, and my first visit home was not until Thanksgiving. I returned an absolute wreck. I was torn, shredded with anxiety; I could hardly sit. I didn't know what was going on. I was terrified of my own level of anxiety.

I began to take glasses from the kitchen. I would wrap them in a towel. Then I would swallow the pieces of glass. I never told anyone until a few years ago. This act was not a communication to anyone else.

I think it was an attempt to make real what it felt like inside of me, to justify feeling so awful. I felt like I was tearing myself up inside. It felt that I was grinding up my very soul. I think that's why I did it, and I don't think I realized it until right now.

Will saw the shape I was in, though he did not know about the glass eating, and had me come in every day, giving up his lunch hour for many days. He insisted that together we could figure out the source of my uncontrollable anxiety.

During a session, I realized that in my mind I wished my mother dead. Then I imagined she had actually died. The anxiety came from my fear that this fantasy could or would kill her, like I had killed my father. As soon as I realized that I had wished her dead, there was this sudden relief. It was a critical breakthrough, and I became a convert to psychotherapy.

I was barely out of this Thanksgiving crisis when I found out the head of Austin Riggs, very famous in world psychiatry, was coming to do a resident training. It was Will's turn, and he asked to present me. Will said, "Look, don't be nervous. This is a test of me, not of you. I will have told them about you before you come in, then this guy will ask you questions, then you leave."

I walked into this board room, a very formal place I'd never been in. There were a lot of men, male psychiatrists, sitting around a large table. I don't think there was another woman in the room. This guy I'd never seen before asked me things like, "Did I see my father in a coffin?" "Did I expect to meet my father in heaven?" Clearly he had a reunion theory that he wanted to prove was the etiology of my suicide stuff. He referred to Gloria at Riggs. He implied that we were probably lesbians. But the questions that upset me the most were about my father.

I walked out of that room, and I was really shook. I said to Will, "Why did he ask me those questions?" I thought those questions were quite cruel.

He answered, "I don't know. If I had been in that position, I wouldn't have." It could have been very tempting for a young resident to make hay of this experience, to try to show off to me. He may have known more than he said, but his answer was very important to me. He stayed on my side. I didn't then have to feel like there was this club of psychiatrists that he was part of, that would judge and exclude me.

After a short visit home for Christmas, I started hemorrhaging the day I returned. Vaginally. It was not properly dealt with; because I had so many somatic complaints, they ignored it. By the time they called Goodman in, I had lost a lot of blood. I went to the infirmary, and things moved quickly.

I remember Goodman came in and said, "God, you have cut yourself repeatedly; you're not going to bleed to death this way." It was incredible how much I bled. There was no medical explanation, just a sudden hormonal imbalance. Although Goodman and I did not talk about it in psyche-soma terms, I think we both knew the timing was no coincidence—I suddenly started to bleed uncontrollably after being home. I believe it was a physical manifestation of my emotional pain.

People from the local hospital came to administer the transfusions. But Goodman wanted to do it himself. Right in front of me, he got terribly annoyed with this doctor because he wanted to do the transfusion. I was tickled by this. "They think that we're not real doctors over here." But it was their blood, and they were going to administer it.

All of this enhanced us a lot. It just made me feel very good. I think I was becoming special to him.

I needed a D&C and went to the local hospital for it. While I was in the hospital, Goodman brought me magazines, sports magazines. He said, "I don't know what kind of magazines you like, so I just got you the kind I would like." I was very touched by that.

Around February, there wasn't a whole hell of a lot to do, and cabin fever set in. I was organizing fun and games on the unit, and Goodman was telling me to cool it. He would say that this was not college. My comeback would be, "Oh, it's a place for crazy people, so you want me to act crazy." I was on report all of the time, but for minor things.

We had a night staff person that nobody liked. She wasn't cruel, but ineffective, pimply, and difficult. One night we surrounded her in the nurses' station and started rhythmically pounding on the glass, which must have just terrified her.

The next day, Goodman just lit into me about being cruel. He said there was no exploring, discussing, or arguing about this. "You can't do that." He had no difficulty giving lectures. [Decent people don't act that way; do you think you are the only person in the world who is in pain?" It was really the moral training I never had.]

Another time I organized a game of running bases. It was a pretty raucous game. Anyway, I threw a ball the length of the ward and threw it badly. It knocked over a lamp next to this woman Betty, a grandmotherly type who was manic depressive. Suddenly she flips out of her depressed state into manic. She's running around the ward very crazy. It was terrifying to me because this was a woman that I really cared about. Fucking up was no big deal, but hurting Betty was. And I was very scared of Goodman's anger once he found out.

I tried to talk to him about it, but I couldn't. He was furious. That was before they had lithium to treat manic depressives, so her flipping into manic was a real problem. There was no choice but to send her down to Carlson I and heavily medicate her with major tranquilizers. Goodman was very protective of all of his patients, and Betty was one of his. I grew more and more frightened that I had destroyed the only relationship that stood between me and my own self-hatred.

I knew that about eight weeks before there had been a successful hanging at Mountain Brook. In my room there was a curved pipe that hung over my bed. Strange that they would have this; it must have been part of the sprinkler system. I took a red shirt, made it into a noose and strung it up over the pipe. I stood on the bed, which was on rollers; once the noose was around my neck, I was going to push the bed out from under me. I was just starting to put this noose around my neck when the bed swung out from the wall, and I fell down between the bed and the wall. I started crying and I cried for five hours without stopping. The noose was still hanging from the pipe when my roommate came in. She freaked out and went screaming down the hall.

Goodman acted very quickly, but I'm sure there was much deliberation before he told me, "I'm sending you down." I pleaded and pleaded. I remember backing up into a corner, like a terrified child or a cornered animal. Once he saw my response, I think it was difficult for him to follow through on it. I said, "If you have to send me down, send me to Carlson I." It was pathetic, I was so frightened. Even to me now, it's heart rending to think of this scene.

He said, "I would if there was a bed, but there is no bed." So I knew that he wasn't just being cruel; again that was confirmed.

They would send this big canvas basket to come in and take away all of your possessions. It came while Goodman was still there. I pleaded, "Well, then send me on visit." That meant you would come back shortly to your own room.

He said, "You can do that for only two days. That's not long enough. I'll visit you every day." He really did everything he could.

So they transferred me to Carlson II. Ice packs were used all the time in seclusion rooms; it was heavy duty. It did not turn out to be as frightening as in my imagination, although it was far from a pleasant place.

He also started me on a drug that was new at the time—Prolixin. It was the latest antipsychotic medication on the market. I got it by injection, and this was a two-week shot. But they didn't know about dosages then; they didn't know about much. I had a very severe reaction to the Prolixin. It made me so restless that literally I could not sit down. The day after I got my first shot I played Ping-Pong for seventeen hours. You can imagine how powerful it was; by the end of two weeks, I was just coming down to the point where I could sit.

Then they'd come to give me another shot. When I saw them, I would try to run away. I was arguing with him, pleading with him to take me off it. I think that he had been so angry about Betty and scared about my suicide attempt that he hadn't really thought it through. The assumption was that the shock treatments had worn off, and so they were trying the Prolixin. In fact, for me it was an interpersonal crisis between him and me.

My mother came to visit me for Easter. She was very helpful with this crisis, the only time she really came to my aide, when she was right and he was wrong. I also think I probably didn't let him forget it. After consultation with his supervisor, they finally took me off the Prolixin.

Although I was on Carlson II only sixteen days, I didn't get my passes back until May. On this very hot day, I took three friends with me to have a picnic. It was one of those freak kind of hot days that you can have in the spring around there. We picked up some beer and wine and went across the Nautilus Bridge—a bridge that spans the Hudson River. We wanted to get to what looked like this very nice beach. But in order to get there, we had to walk through this muck, with the most awful stench.

On the way back, I decided that I did not want to walk through this muck again. I thought it was just too disgusting.

So I decided to swim across the Hudson. This other young woman, girl, decided that she would come with me. The friends who were with us took our shoes and socks. The water temperature was very cold. We jumped into the water and Jennifer, who was not as strong a swimmer as I was, got caught in this very quick current. She headed downstream and I thought I was watching her drown. I screamed to her not to panic, but the noise of the river was so great out there. She got caught right under the bridge, which made the current just that much swifter. I kept screaming at her to relax. I figured as long as she didn't panic she would eventually land someplace that was safe.

Before I got swept under the bridge, I came to one of the pilings, and the force of the water, particularly in spring, was tremendous. I made my way to a wide part of the river, where the water parted. There was no current, so I could just sit. I was frightened and then frightened for Jennifer. Once again, here I was responsible for killing somebody, because of my lack of judgment.

We both made it across. There were some men working on the electrical wires who called the police when they saw us. The police came, asked us all kinds of questions, and took us back to Mountain Brook.

There was a message waiting for me that Goodman wanted to see me as soon as I changed. I knew that I was in for it—big time. I had done a pretty stupid thing, but it was not some kind of deliberate acting out. I just hadn't calculated the current of the river and I hadn't calculated the fact that it was severely polluted.

Goodman said that it was very stupid. He called poison control to find out what injections we needed. We got more injections than if we were traveling through Africa. He said, "You know the only thing that gives me any satisfaction is the image of how many needles you'll have to sustain." He was really ripped, but his anger did not bother me because it was always loving. We were fighting, but we weren't at risk of alienation.

About this time, my mother told Goodman that the money was running out. Mountain Brook was expensive, very expensive, something like $30,000 a year back then. She appealed to my grandparents, and they said to send me to a state hospital.

I was devastated when Goodman told me that I would have to leave. I accused him of not having advocated enough for me. I started threatening everything. I said I was going to get some carbolic acid from the hardware store across the street and drink it, or jump off the Nautilus Bridge. I was so distraught; I knew I was not ready to go.

I think he really tried to make himself believe that I was ready, that I could make it. I said, "What can I do? I'm not prepared to do anything."

He said, "What do girls your age do?"

"I guess they go to college or work. I can't do that. Where can I live?"

Goodman said that I couldn't live at home. I was reduced to being a terrified child again. I was being abandoned in a most profound way. I even started having some dissociative states where I wouldn't know where I was. I think the glass eating went up, but I didn't tell anybody. I was getting real desperate again because I knew that I wasn't OK.

Goodman said that all these threats frightened him. He said that if I continued, he would have no choice but to send me to a state institution. I knew that if I went there, there would be no therapy. [Therapy had now become very important to me. I understood that it worked to make me feel better. How separate therapy was from Will Goodman at that point was hard to know. So I silenced those threats.

In our last sessions, he talked to me about loving me. That wasn't going to change because of the distance. It did not feel like something that he would routinely say or something that was easy for him to say. Somewhere along the way, because of my history of sexual abuse, he explicitly said that his love would never become sexual. It was a comfort to me that he had said that.

I arrived home. There seemed to be no choice about that, and I was morose, depressed, frightened, and anxious. I was lonely. Most of my friends were in jobs or college or just engaged in other lives. My only friends were those who were in institutions.

And I went back in therapy with Jameson, which was a problem.

My mother introduced me to a resident at Roosevelt Hospital. She knew his family, and I went out on a date with him. He was very big, and he was very compelling to me. I went up to his room for a drink before dinner, and he raped me. He got up, went into the bathroom, and cleaned up; he came back out, and he apologized. I went out for dinner with him, but the whole dinner I was trying to remember if I knew where my car was, if I knew how to get out of New York City. I had probably driven in and out of the city more than two hundred times in my life, but I was clearly very disorganized by this experience. I was ashamed and felt responsible for what happened.

When I told Jameson about this—the psychiatrist who told me that I dressed in a sexless way and wondered why I avoided contact with men—he told me that I was responsible for what happened. I was sure that he was right.

I think that's when I began to cook how I would kill myself.

Part of the illness is an absolute foreclosure of options. There is no way to see that there is another therapist in the world, that I could advocate for myself, or that everything Jameson said was not true.

I was beginning to drink, and I would drink a great deal before sessions, but I don't think he noticed. I would tell him that my life was miserable, everything was so meaningless. But since I had a job at NYU and was living on my own—I had gotten an apartment—he would say, "That's terrific." It wasn't reassuring; he wasn't listening. He was screening out my reality and replacing it with the rosy picture he wanted to see. I got more and more desperate with this.

I asked Jameson for a sleeping pill prescription. After I just battered him, he finally gave me a prescription for five Tuinol. That night, I very carefully forged the prescription.

The next day, I went to work with the prescription tucked in my pocket. But I lost it. To give you a sense of the pitch of things and how desperate I was, I went rifling through garbage cans on Broadway, the bag ladies eyeing me the whole time. Finally, I went back to the place where I had taken my tea break. I hurried over to this pile of rubbish in a corner that they were just about to sweep away, and noticed there was one piece of white paper. I had found my prescription, and I was just elated. At the drug store, I distracted the pharmacist so he would not call Jameson.

My new roommate of four days told me she would be studying at the library until 11:00. At about 7:30, I took ten of the pills. I was terrified. To medicate the terror, to continue with the act, I took the remaining thirty pills. It was a lethal dose. I was very stoned; just before passing out, I called Jameson. He told me to call him back in ten minutes.

My roommate just happened to return early to get a book. Jameson called. She said, "Lindsey doesn't want to talk with you. She's sobbing." The sobbing was actually my gasping for breath.

He called an ambulance, and they took me to the hospital. I was unconscious for three days. Later I spoke with the emergency room doctor, who said that when I came in it was touch and go. Apparently they weren't at all sure that I was going to survive.

When I came to, I was still high. But once I came down from the drug, I was left feeling only despair and emptiness. I was angry that I had not succeeded. I just wanted to be dead. There was no relief in being alive.

They decided that I had to go back into another long-term

institution, and somehow there was money available for my care. They would not send me back to Mountain Brook, however. Now that I'm working in these places, I know how professionals often process this stuff. They may have thought that I was simply trying to get back into Mountain Brook. But this suicide attempt was truly lethal; it was not a gesture. I mean I knew how to do that, too, and this was not a gesture.

They sent me to the Adolescent Treatment Center, ATC, which was experimental, sponsored by a very famous hospital in New York. This place was very bizarre. In every way that it could be different from Mountain Brook, it was. It was unstructured. There were extraordinary levels of acting out, breakage, drunkenness, running away. The competition over who was the sickest was intense.

One woman got admitted because her "symptom" was prostitution. She brought her tricks to the center. One of the kids there jumped in front of a subway. He was not killed, but he lost both his legs. My best friend there was a wonderful young man named Tim. He committed suicide shortly after leaving the place.

Clearly there was a lot of evidence that I was a prime therapy candidate. They did not understand treatment. I don't know anybody who got better there. I had a therapist, a foreign psychiatrist with little command of English, who misunderstood my name. So for the first three months—I was there nine months—he called me Linseed. During our first interview, he said that when I got severely anxious, instead of hurting myself or breaking something, I should use this. He then handed me a child's whistle, a plastic red whistle, on a rope. I was bemused, stunned, embarrassed but mostly frightened that a person who thought this way was to be in charge of my care.

One of my roommates there, a very disturbed young woman, was married. Her husband, Stephen, came to visit her, but she was restricted. Somehow he found the window of the room we were in. The window, unlike many hospitals I was in, opened, but just a very small crack, so that only the thinnest of people could escape. So he talked through this crack to Candy. Since she was not allowed to leave the unit and I was, I went out to find him. I then told him that he didn't need to worry about sneaking around trying to see her; he should just assert his rights.

I don't think Candy was there more than two or three weeks. She was very disturbed, but Stephen wasn't getting any help from her family, and he just couldn't afford to keep her there. After she left, I started to go and visit them, which was about an hour away. It was, of course, totally illegal. We all got off on that.

Since everything was initiated by acting out, my whole level of acting out really skyrocketed. In response, they drugged me very, very heavily. I went from one injection of sodium amytal, 700 milligrams every four hours—which is enough to make an elephant sleepy—to 1200 milligrams of thorazine. I walked around like a zombie until I got used to it. I stopped eating. I remember one time during a therapy session, I was supposed to eat in front of my psychiatrist. I did what a little child would do: I stuffed the mashed potatoes, peas, and chicken under the cushions when he wasn't looking. I was twenty-three years old.

This place was just awful. But I did receive some help from two men there. One was an aide, the other a nurse. I got to such a place of infantile regression that I may have gotten it out of my system forever. I played out everything. But the not eating became serious. I just willed this, and for three months I did not eat. They tried to force-feed me, which was a very unpleasant battle.

At one point, I distracted the person who was watching me one on one, ran to a window, and smashed it, badly lacerating my arm. The director of the place just happened to be walking under the window at the time.

They sent me to Gracie Square Hospital, which is a rich person's Bellevue. I was put on a medical unit. I thought they were cruel there. The place I had just left, with all of its faults—and there were many—had some warmth. There was some real warmth to the people there. Here they were cold and constantly annoyed by the patients they were supposed to care for.

I would unscrew light bulbs and break them, then eat the slivers. At one point, I practically ate a whole glass. A nurse walked in while I was eating one of the pieces. They got very excited at this, took X-rays, and ran tests, but there was nothing they could do. A surgeon came in, a very sadistic guy, described how I would die. He told me that as my digestive system attempted to digest the glass, my gizzards would be ripped to shreds, and I would bleed to death.

But I didn't. Other than abdominal pain, I don't know that I ever suffered physically from the glass eating.

I had my first true psychotic break there. I was completely out of it; I didn't know where I was. I thought I was in a bowling alley.

I still wasn't eating. I was on IV's. I was severely malnourished, but I wasn't losing a lot of weight because I was impacted. My system was becoming extremely toxic.

A nurse there said, "You can't eat oatmeal, or applesauce, but you can eat glass." Anyway, I started to eat, gained a little weight, and they sent me back to ATC.

Slowly, I think I had just had enough of that place. I wanted to get out. After about eight or nine months, I left there.

I moved back to the same apartment and moved back into the relationship with Jameson for a short while.

Stephen, Candy's husband, came to visit me. Stephen had left her after she tried to castrate him while he lay sleeping one night. He was down looking for a place to live, a new job, and a new start in New York. His life was in ragged disrepair; he was trying to work and raise an infant as a single parent. We really just hung out as friends. I was too gonzo to consider it a romance, but I was growing to like him a lot.

My mother was attempting to facilitate the relationship, I think because she was desperate not to have sole responsibility for me, and also because she liked Stephen very much. She had strong moral standards, but she arranged two different trips, one to Florida and one skiing, while he was still married. She put a lot of subtle, persistent pressure on me and, I think, to some extent on him to consummate the relationship.

But all was not sweetness and light.

There were hundreds of different episodes, but this is perhaps the most freaky. This still upsets Stephen—to think that I could have done this while he was in the next room. I was in my apartment; I stood in front of the mirror, and I wanted to completely disfigure my face] I looked at my face in the mirror, picked up a glass, and smashed it, full force, into my face. At the very last moment, I shifted the focus of the blow, and I totally split open my forehead. The blood was pouring out. It was a terrible wound.

The police took me to the hospital. I remember this cop was sweating, he was trying to hold my forehead together. He was very nervous about the amount of blood I was losing. Again I was in extraordinary conflict because I knew he was being so kind to me because he thought it was an accident—I told him I fell. He had no idea I did it to myself. But I knew.

I got some excellent plastic surgery, but I still have a fairly significant scar on my forehead.

Jameson didn't believe that I fell, but I never told him the truth.

Shortly after this, he told me he could no longer treat me. Jason Gold, who was the head of Riverview Hospital—was back in Riverview—and who had been the first person to convince my mother I needed help, said to me that I was running out of options. Psychiatrists, therapists, did not want to work with me because I was considered too big a risk. Finally, Novick, the psychiatrist, agreed to see me.

Stephen was visiting me everyday, but there were days on end where I was so out of it, I did not even know if he had been there or not. It was a difficult time for him, too. He'd been fired from his job, his baby was in foster care, and his wife was insane. He was feeling very down.

One evening, Stephen went to a neighborhood bar and got himself pretty looped. He left the bar, bought some flowers and attempted to deliver them to the ward about midnight. When he got there, they refused to allow the flowers to come in because of the lateness of the hour.

Undaunted, Stephen went across the street where a new wing of the hospital was under construction. He knew that the window of my room in seclusion was connected to the new wing being constructed.

He sneaked past the night watchman and climbed up the stairs that were built. I was on the eighth floor, but the stairs only went as far as the third floor. He then took a ladder to each subsequent floor, climbed up, then pulled the ladder up after himself. He made it to the seventh floor, where there was the beginning of a passageway to connect the two buildings. He climbed up onto the roof of the passageway and then put the ladder against the wall, right under the window of the seclusion room. He climbed up the ladder and managed to get within a few feet of my room. It was probably one o'clock in the morning by now, and I'm sure he was wildly drunk, balancing on girders eight stories high with a bouquet of flowers in his hand. This was New York City—someone sees you on the rooftop, you can get shot.

I'm in the seclusion room, as usual not sleeping, and I hear my name being called, "Lindsey," "Lindsey," "Lindsey." I keep hearing it and I go to the attendant, who is half asleep.

I tell him, "Someone is calling my name."

He says, "Oh, go to bed. You're having a hallucination."

Stephen had no choice but to go back down, pulling the ladder after him. He sneaked past the night watchman again and left the flowers at the door of the hospital.

There was romance, but I'm not sure what kind of stories they'll make to tell our grandchildren.

I was quite psychotic during this stay. Again, I believe it was related to my not eating. During one episode, I thought I was watching myself do a swan dive. Actually, what I did was stand on the top of the bed, hold my hands behind my back, and dive headfirst onto the tile floor. I knocked myself out. Several hours later, I woke up strapped to a stretcher. I was just flipping further and further out. The only person that I could see from my gurney was a very old lady who was being fed through tubes in her nostrils. I knew they were getting desperate about my not eating, and so I assumed that this very old lady was me. I began to believe that's who I was.

Guess who walks in the door? Jameson. Guess whose patient this eighty-five-year-old woman is? Jameson's. I'm now completely convinced that this woman is me. He stops by the stretcher—I'm restrained—he says to me, "Fancy meeting you here," or something equally absurd. "What are you doing here?"

I said, "I'm senile."

He said, "How old are you?"

I said, "Twenty-five."

He said, "I think you're a little young to be senile." And he walks up to the old lady, absolutely confirming my belief that I was in fact her. At this point, I completely believed that I would never be out of the hospital again.

I don't remember bathing. I was in my blue jeans for days and days and days. I think they had given up on trying to get me to change. I would sleep in them. I was psychotic. One day a new patient came on the floor who had been a psychiatrist at Mountain Brook when I was there, a young resident who I had liked very much. That really flipped me out. I couldn't keep track of my reality.

I decided one morning that I would get out of seclusion. I made a goal for myself to stay out for two hours. At that point, they weren't keeping me there; I was so frightened, they couldn't get me out.

I left the seclusion area, and I was sitting with a group of hospital friends. Celeste, a woman who was manic depressive, would tell me what went on with me when I was too out of it to know. She said that the sounds that came out of me were like a pig about to be slaughtered. She said they were the most horrible sounds she had ever heard out of any human being.

Suddenly all these doctors came by and walked through these big doors onto the ward. In terror, I ran and pounded on the seclusion door to get back in. They were setting up for shock treatment, and they were annoyed. I was back, and they were annoyed. I turned to go into my room, and there was a little old man standing next to me totally naked. I had never seen him before. I screamed, and the nurse there made fun of me, "Well, have you never seen a naked man before?"

I was fighting off the need to hallucinate. It was almost orgasmic, not in the sense of anything pleasurable, but it was just as forceful. It was like a biological need, it was that strong. And that's the best explanation I can give to someone who has not been through this. I remember trying to keep it at bay until I felt I was in a safe place to do it.

There was an aide named Russell, a spectacular older black man who was just wonderful to me. He saw the shape I was in. He put this naked man somewhere else, and he said, "I'm sorry, Lindsey. We were just getting this man ready for shock treatment, so you can't go into your room now."

Russell found this other room for me. He knew something was going on with me and that I needed to be alone. He shut the door. I started into this hallucination. My body and head were separating. My head stayed on the pillow while my body floated above my head, truncating and turning into smoke. The psychiatrist, Novick, came into my room and said, "I want you to tell me exactly what's going on." And I did. He said, "That's not a hallucination, that's a delusion," which is not accurate, but that's what he said. He asked, "Do you want to go home?"

I snapped. I was out of the psychosis. I was going home. He just totally changed the reality. Then I went into this full-blown manic stage. I was zooming.

I was crying and laughing alternately. I showered, I washed my hair. There were so many rat's nests in my hair it took Celeste two hours to comb it out. When Novick saw all this, he decided he would have me go out on visits rather than discharging me immediately. I started going home during the day and came back to the hospital at night, which was a fairly good plan.

I think I said to myself that I had done everything that crazy people do. There was really nothing left in the repertoire of being crazy that I had not experienced. Clearly I was far from being well, but that experience was over.

I was discharged from the hospital, but physically I was in pretty critical shape. I was now eighty-four pounds, and Novick said that if I lost three more pounds I would die. I looked like an Auschwitz survivor. I could not sit like people sit because I was on bone. So it seemed like I was through being crazy, but now I was going to die. Novick took me off the medication. He said, "They're telling me that if I take you off this medication you'll kill yourself." The last time they took me off it I had eaten all this glass. "But if you stay on it, you're going to die."

So he took me off everything. They sent me for a swallowing test at Mount Sinai and found out that I had reverse peristalsis. I could chew with difficulty, but everything that I swallowed would come back out of my mouth. I started taking phenothiazines for it.

I went home. I gained weight, but I was in a pretty severe depression.

My first Sunday home, Stephen packed a picnic lunch, took me out on the Hudson, and proposed marriage. My response to his proposal was, "You're out of your fucking mind." I told him, "I don't understand your wanting to marry me after you have finally freed yourself from a relationship with this other crazy person."

I think I was both relieved and insulted by his answer. "Compared to her, you are a third-class neurotic." I believe that Stephen always saw my potential for health.

Getting married was a natural act. I loved Stephen. I don't think that my ability to love was ever at base impaired.

I also felt that I had a debt to my mother. She had been injured by me greatly, and I needed to do something about that. Getting married to Stephen was recompense to her.

I was trying to raise a child and was about as well equipped to do this as a young child. In fact, it alleviated a lot of my guilt when a therapist I was seeing said, "Here you are, trying to raise a child, and you're no more than a child yourself."

It was a rough time. I would look out the window. I would see people going to work. I would look at them and think they were miraculous. Stephen was shouldering all the domestic tasks during this time.

I saw two movies that had impact. In *Night of the Iguana*, there is this scene where a defrocked priest, Richard Burton, is going through the DTs. Two important conversations go on that night. One is with a spinster woman who has been traveling all over the world with her elderly father. This defrocked priest asks if she ever had a sexual experience. She says only one: She let some gondolier hold her underwear. He says, "That's disgusting." I remember hearing from her, "Nothing human is disgusting." I had always felt disgusting. To think, to imagine, to play with the idea that "nothing human is disgusting" was wonderful.

Later in this movie, Ava Gardner is talking to Richard Burton trying to help him get through the night. She says to him, "The goal of life is to survive." I thought, my God, I had done that. It was the first sense I had that I had done something right, that I'd done enough. I think that began to turn the depression around.

The next week I saw *Suddenly Last Summer*. It's a movie about how families can drive their children crazy. Even though I had discussed my parents, my family, at length in therapy, I really believed, I knew, the problems were my fault. My core was somehow defective. The real crazy person in the movie was the mother, but the daughter was manifesting the symptoms; she was the one who looked insane to the rest of the world. I felt, "Oh my God."

Things started to open up. The depression was beginning to give way.

I went back to school. I found a good therapist. I rapidly got involved in the political scene in 1968. I knew that I would never be in a hospital again. Other than in my dreams, or to visit, I never have.

LINDSEY'S REFLECTIONS ABOUT HER EXPERIENCE

[Lindsey is in a unique position to comment about her remarkable recovery. She was in psychotherapy for eighteen years trying to understand, and through the process of understanding, promote her emotional well-being. Lindsey herself now works as a psychotherapist and administrator of a program for seriously disturbed individuals. Her emotional and intellectual familiarity with the healing process is truly intimate.]

Sometimes I wonder: How sick was I? I question whether I was a fraud and it was all an effort to gain attention. In our culture, since there is no tumor, no blood test to prove its existence, we sometimes assume mental illness is not real. A very dear friend who is a therapist and knows much of my history helped with this. She said to me, "I don't know what your definition is of crazy, but anyone who would go to such extraordinary lengths to gain attention or establish a relationship is pretty crazy."

The time I nearly bled to death, when I started to hemorrhage spontaneously, was almost a relief. It was something concrete for me and others to witness. After visiting home, I had so much pain it just had to be expressed. I think this particular time, since the amount of rage and pain was so great and the emotional outlet was not sufficient, bleeding was a way for my body to express it.

Cutting is more than an indicator to a blind other world that you're in big trouble. It helps to focus the pain in a manageable way. The physical pain from cutting yourself is minor; it's superficial. It focuses the pain and makes it comprehensible. Emotional pain is different; it's so diverse and so all-encompassing that it's beyond understanding. I get a sense that the primitive thinking behind cutting is comparable to bloodletting—it draws out the toxin temporarily.

Others sometimes would say to me, "Look at all the nice things that go on in your life. Cheer up." But that just made me feel worse—I shouldn't be this fucked up, I shouldn't be sick. My favorite was, "Look at all the suffering of other people." Since I was someone who had no barrier, no skin between my suffering and that of others, that one really helped me an enormous amount. I never understood that as a tactic. I guess the belief was that some kinds of suffering—starving or serious illness—are real, whereas mine could just be stopped, if I only believed in God or tried harder or loved my parents.

Willfulness was a thread woven throughout the process of my recovery. Will was very important but not something that I can just pull out and examine. I only remember one moment of conscious willfulness: I decided I was going to leave the seclusion room for two hours. I assume there were more moments like that. But I didn't think of them as courageous. I was the scum of the earth, and I should be dead. I was a coward for staying alive.

I think the Tennessee Williams movies helped because they made me recognize that perhaps there really was something courageous about my daring to live when I felt like scum.

I would like to find Novick and ask him about his intervention: "Do you want to go home?" Where did it come from? I mean one in a million therapists would have said something like that. He comes walking in on the middle of a full-blown psychotic hallucination. It was genius or luck, I don't know.

I hesitate to use this expression, but it was like shock therapy. He intervened when I was most crazy and just totally normalized it. He named it something different from what it was. For it was a hallucination, not a delusion. Every belief system I had that was feeding the psychosis was gone, shot to hell. Suddenly, my reality was very different. I mean it wasn't rosy, but it was different, and my behavior changed dramatically. I became manic, and five hours later I went home to visit, scaring everybody because my moods were so weird. The manic stuff started to resolve itself, I think, because I felt I was done being crazy. I had lived this experience to the hilt, there was nothing new to be learned.

I then went into a depression for a good three months. I think I was depressed then because I knew that I was done as a mental patient. I could no longer take refuge in being crazy. For me, a psych ward was home; it was the only hearth that I really had. In a sense, it meant that I could never go home again. I think, every once in a while when I'm talking about this, of my poor mother. Were she ever to hear this, how shocking and horrifying it would be to her.

Like my experience with Novick, health can come from strange places. Breakthroughs will happen when they're not expected. I remember one incident. There was this kid—this pimply, English, catatonic boy. He had a private room, and having one was envied by everybody. All the patients, about thirty-five of us, had to eat in this tiny dining room. We were so jammed in there, and there were constant scenes. One time a very large woman had a grand mal seizure. She threw the entire table over; food was flying into people's faces. This very sardonic guy who was sitting next to me said, without flinching, without cracking a smile, "The food's bad, but not that bad."

Anyway, this catatonic kid for some reason did not have to sit in the dining room. I resented him, and I'm sure I reflected the resentment of a lot of people. Everybody was grumbling about him, but nobody was doing anything. He just annoyed the hell out of me as he stood on the edge of this room and looked so superior—this kid who was probably so miserable.

So I took off at top speed from one end of the hall and tackled him. He went flying in the air, but he came down on top of me and started flailing away with his fists. He was really hitting me hard. I mean I can almost feel it on my back now. He was screaming. He hadn't talked in a year, and now he was screaming all this foul language. It was something; the nurses wanted to kill me, and it was probably one of the times they put me in seclusion. It was a big scene.

He got discharged. Later on, while I was walking the ward, his resident came up to me, and he said, "You promise me that you will never tell anybody what I'm about to tell you?" I promised. He said, "I don't think that anything could have helped him more. He's moving about, talking all the time now." It was a tremendous cathartic release for him, like Novick's moment with me. I had no altruistic motives whatsoever; I was being hostile, but this kid got better.

There's really nothing abstract about the desire to stay alive. It comes from an attachment and connection with other human beings. When I tackled this kid, though it wasn't the kind of connection we usually hope for, he did reconnect with the world. Some people may want to live because of an attachment to God, or to nature, or to animals. But for most of us, that's not enough. It has to be people or another person. That's what makes you want to live. That's what heals you.

Love has a great deal to do with my recovery. As a child, I was loved by my mother and father, there is no question. I was loved, however, in a sievelike way. They could not love beyond their own narcissism; I was an extension of them.

My relationship with Goodman was not an enmeshed love. His boundaries were always clear. He did love me, though he may use a very different language than I do, and I definitely loved him. One of our major discussions and, at times, arguments was whether the love was transferential or real. Within the past few years, we have both grown sophisticated enough to give up these distinctions, to recognize that probably all love is in good part transferential.

I internalized and held on to Goodman long after I stopped seeing him. His presence in my life contradicted every other message—that I was hopeless, that I was worthless, that I was a murderer, that I was a seductress, immoral, crazy, that I was beyond redemption.

I read about a little boy who defeated his brain tumor by visualizing space ships that shot at and destroyed his cancer. My analogous process was visualizing Goodman, bringing him to mind. For the boy with cancer, spaceships were his metaphor. For me it was this loving, controlling, authoritarian, absolutely protective father.

It's funny. There are two reasons why I need to stay anonymous. The first is the very real prejudice in the profession against people with histories like mine doing psychotherapy. The other is the way I describe my work as a psychotherapist. I don't think about treatment in terms of cure; I think about what will make love possible. When people ask, "How do you work?" I won't mention this. I will talk in terms of psychodynamic phenomena. That's how unappreciated this kind of thinking is in our profession. I could probably be hung for this, but I think in terms of love—of working through the terrible shame that got you sick, the shame of being sick, the forgiveness of

<u>people who wrought such hell in your life and the forgiveness of</u>
<u>yourself. This allows love.</u>

Twenty-five years after her stay at Mountain Brook, Lindsey's relationship with her former therapist, Dr. William Goodman, is still significant. Though she never reentered treatment with him, she writes or visits him a couple of times a year.

Dr. Goodman today is clinical director of Mountain Brook, one of the most respected psychiatric hospitals in the United States. When I asked Dr. Goodman if he would meet with me in the hope of better understanding Lindsey's illness and recovery, he agreed. But he agreed only if Lindsey were also present. The issues of confidentiality and trust are sacred to him; he wanted to make sure there would be no misunderstandings, no violation of trust.

Before meeting with Dr. Goodman, Lindsey showed me around Mountain Brook. As a psychologist, I've served my time in mental hospitals. But my familiarity is mostly with state hospitals, or, in Lindscy's words, "the snake pit variety." Mountain Brook looked like an expensive eastern college: beautiful grounds with brick buildings that did not have quite enough room between them to present either their strength or grace. She pointed out renovated buildings that used to be Carlson I and Carlson II and the formal boardroom where intern trainings were once conducted.

Will Goodman greeted Lindsey with a hug and made me feel welcome as we shook hands. Besides knowing Lindsey's feelings about Will, the psychotherapists' grapevine yielded only high praise for the man and his work. He is known to be human, humble, and tough. Despite the high expectations, I found his warmth and utter realness surprising.

Lindsey seemed very comfortable as Will began talking about her illness and stay at Mountain Brook. Though my presence added a slight wrinkle, the terrain was familiar for the two of them. Over the years, they have spent many hours trying to understand Lindsey's illness, the reasons for her health, and the nature of their relationship.

REFLECTIONS OF WILLIAM GOODMAN, M.D.

In a sense, Lindsey and I were colleagues. I never felt that I was the all-knowing psychiatrist. All Lindsey had to do was give me some associations, and I would make the connections. At the time, I was a young man, relatively inexperienced in both medicine and psychiatry. Maybe it would have been tougher if I had more experience and thought I knew more than I did. It was natural for me to say, "I've got a little more experience and knowledge about this, but we're really working together to solve something that's very important," though I'm sure at times I sounded like I came out of a textbook or something I'd read in *Reader's Digest* the night before.

Lindsey was dealing with a very malignant process. It was worrisome, very worrisome, puzzling, I wasn't sure how it would turn out, but I don't think I saw it as lethal. I never expected her to be seriously impaired. This belief is not based upon the facts because her process was very malignant, no question about that. It had to do with who Lindsey was.

What was it about Lindsey that made her different? Determination. Even when she was most despondent or angry or both, the drive was always there. She never quite gave up. Each time I saw Lindsey, I felt that there was going to be some kind of activity, some sort of movement.

I can contrast these qualities with a number of other patients I work with who do not seem as disturbed in the way they think about things or their behaviors. But they also don't have this strong drive, this desire to understand, to interact with and impact upon others.

Lindsey is obviously intelligent. But there are a lot of intelligent people. What she has is a highly developed ability to make connections and an intense intellectual curiosity to learn and discover about herself. She couldn't stop being that way; it was a struggle that she could not let go of, so I think it forced her to come to terms with her life.

As you know, Lindsey had some very difficult occurrences in her life. They were not simple tragedies or threats; her worldview was much more complex. She was continually dealing with them in a way that at times exhausted her and those around her.

There were reasons why she and I got off on the same foot. Lindsey was clearly in a lot of pain over the loss of her father. Just before she was admitted, I lost my brother to an automobile accident. This was a brother with whom I was extremely close. I guess most brothers are close, but we grew up doing everything together, hiking in Yellowstone, playing ball together. It wasn't conceivable at that point in my life that something like that could happen to me, something that challenging to my stability.

When I returned from Iowa, Lindsey was my next patient. You might think that I would not be as open or fully present because I was trying to deal with my loss, with the grieving. But I think in some ways I was more fully present, more alive, more curious to see how Lindsey was handling her process while I was handling mine.

You could talk about this in terms of some kind of psychiatric theory, but, to be honest, I think Lindsey tapped into the kind of person I am.

Sometimes my approach is not too cushioned. I think I'm fairly direct. I'm fairly honest. Like Lindsey, I want to understand myself and my world. I try not to fool myself about too many things—including myself. That has been helpful to me as a psychiatrist. Patients will forgive you for much. They will not forgive you for trying to be what you're not.

As I've gotten older, I'm more comfortable being myself and not as worried about a technique. But at that time, I tried to be more nonrevealing, to act as I thought a psychiatrist was supposed to act. There were a lot of temptations after a year of psychotherapy to try and walk like and talk like a Freudian. I was more myself with Lindsey than with other patients, which I think had more to do with her than with me. Lindsey sure could read who I was at a particular moment. She knew when I was angry or when I was concerned. She really did. I think that was helpful to therapy, to her and to me.

Many of my interventions had little to do with my education in psychiatry and much more to do with my growing up in Indiana at the knee of two country doctors and a country nurse. My grandfather practiced fifty-seven years and Dad for forty-two. My mother was a country nurse. They had very strong beliefs about what was right and what was wrong, that limits needed to be set. Lindsey brought that out more, required that more than other patients who were not as challenging.

At points, the interaction was very strong. I'm sure in ways it was reassuring but at other times [Will turns to Lindsey] you must've said, "Well, I know he cares, but if he goes after me this way, he can't understand." I think there was part of you that always sensed I did understand.

I am very possessive of my own patients, my own family, and my own self. Years ago, I went fishing with my son on the Potomac. He was about five, and he fell in. I jumped in, and I grabbed him by his belt and pulled him out. He looked at me, and he said, "You saved my life," which was a bit dramatic. As a young adult, when I thought he was in trouble in Houston, I said, "Listen, Ed, I didn't haul your ass out of the Potomac to lose it in Texas." It was the same kind of feeling with Lindsey.

[Will directs his attention to Lindsey again.] There were very powerful things that were destroying or messing you up, and I think I was basically saying, at times, speaking to your unconscious, "This is not going to happen." Lindsey understood so much; she understood more or sensed more about me in some ways than I did. I think I almost counted on that. The message was "God damn it, Lindsey, you know what you are doing, and you don't do this."

Lindsey would look at me in genuine anger or horror and say, "Why are you beating up on me for this. I don't know what I'm doing." My response at some level was, "Well, if you don't know, then you should know. You are not going to do that. Cut it out. You don't swim out in the middle of the Hudson River and go under."

The kind of trust Lindsey had in me resonates. That brings out something good in you. She brought out an awareness that I was very appreciative of. It wasn't always easy. She would not let me get by with less than a full response. I was asking her to face certain things, and in some ways she was asking the same of me. Not to smooth over feelings with platitudes or easy explanations. She would not let me do that, and I am grateful to her for that. It was a good patient relationship, but it was much more than that—it was a good person encounter.

I've seen a number of explanations of how this kind of love or bonding can produce biochemical and physiological changes in the body. I'm sure that's true, but I'm not sure that the transformation of the emotional into the biological is satisfactory. There's no question that patients with "fatal" biological illnesses who, if you can put it under one rubric, have a reason to live, generally do much better. I have a few patients with a very serious thinking disorder, schizophrenia, who nonetheless live with it well. Yet there are other patients with diagnoses not nearly as serious who are tremendously impaired by their illness. If you've got a reason to live and a person to share that with, it makes a difference.

Lindsey taught me a great deal. Our interaction did. I do not think that I would be the psychiatrist I am today, good or bad, had I not treated Lindsey. I'm sure of that.

[After talking with Dr. Goodman for more than an hour, it became apparent that the relationship between Will Goodman and Lindsey Reynolds was a loving one. I shared this feeling with both of them.]

Will Goodman: I resisted using that language because of the obvious erotic components to it. I said to Lindsey that I did not want there to be any misunderstandings. Lindsey wrote me a few letters trying to straighten me out on that, too. She said that there can be a loving relationship, which obviously there is, without a violation of the therapist/patient relationship. Basically she said not to be so God damn scared of it! [He turns to Lindsey.] I know that may be an offense to your syntax and your way with words, but that was essentially it.

Lindsey Reynolds: I just think that you're funny. There are ways that you are so male—the way that you talk about love. I know how much you love me, and I know how much I love you. It's there. You tend to put it aside just a little bit.

When we ended, when I left Mountain Brook, you hugged me warmly. I was just a kid then, and you talked about loving me. You and I have tried to analyze it. I know that there are all of these psychic and psychodynamic realities. But I think it comes down to this. When I came here my belief was that I had a dog that loved me. Remember Tracey?

Will: Yea.

Lindsey: When I left here, I had another. . .

Will: Dog?

Lindsey: I had a person who loved me.

Will: You know, because I don't know how to express it, without getting all tangled up in it, doesn't mean, as you well know, that it isn't there.

You call it "so male." I'm not sure it's tied to that as much as it is tied to the way this male grew up.

Our family never hugged one another until my brother died. We would always shake hands. So I learned that way. It wasn't too hard for me to express my feelings of care or love verbally. When I got the call July 12, and Larry Nash drove me to the airport at 2:00 A.M. . . . [He turns away from Lindsey to speak to me.]

Parenthetically, it ticked me off that she thought Larry was so suave, good-looking, eastern, and Will, the midwestern hick. She said, "God, at least I could have gotten a psychiatrist that was good-looking." I'm sure she thought—who in the hell have I gotten hooked up with?

But, anyway, when I got off the plane, Dad and Mom were there. Dad came into my arms crying. That was the first time we ever hugged; it just wasn't done.

So when I hugged you, Lindsey, it really meant something.

Lindsey: I knew how you felt about me, and it made a difference. When I took those Tuinol for this very carefully planned death, when I called Jameson, which is the only thing that saved my life, from what I can tell, I know that it just wasn't Jameson I was calling. I knew that you loved me, and it felt unconditional. I did not have to be anything or do anything. You loved me for who I was, and that's what held at the darkest moments.

WALTER PURINGTON

In the beginner's mind there are many possibilities, but in the expert's there are few.

Shunryu Suzuki,
Zen Mind, Beginner's Mind

When I called to arrange the interview with Walter Purington, he answered the phone breathing heavily. I assumed his labored breathing was a result of his cancer or a side effect of treatment. But I was wrong. Walter was out of breath because he had run in from outside to get the phone. He had been in the backyard chopping wood.

Walter's diagnosis of meningeal carcinomatosis, established at a regional hospital, was confirmed by a national expert at Duke University. Walter's oncologist wrote that his chances of staying alive for three years were 1 in 1,000. A second physician estimated the probability as even more remote. He said the chances of Walter's surviving even a year were 1 in 1,000.

Walter received radiation therapy, but only because he insisted upon it. His doctors did not think that any kind of treatment could help. In fact, according to the note I received from his physician: "Following the completion of radiation therapy, the patient returned home with a poor prognosis. He was referred to a hospice for terminal care and an acupuncturist for treatment of pain."

The Puringtons live in a remote section of a small rural town. Walter and his wife, Lillian, welcomed me warmly into their home. Their eldest daughter was preparing supper while their two youngest children watched television. During my visit, the whole family focused—they almost seemed to hover—about Walter.

He and I sat at the kitchen table, for our interview. He was tall and gangly, about 55, with brown hair giving way to gray and a light complexion. He wore a red flannel shirt, blue jeans, and heavy work boots. It was hard work getting him to talk; he was slow and plodding in response to questions. He obviously could speak his mind—he just didn't have much need to. Lillian joined us for most of the interview. Her physical and emotional solidness was especially striking. Although Lillian's style was less deliberate than Walter's, she usually deferred to her husband before answering.

I found myself treading lightly in this initial interview, for only eighteen months had passed since Walter's highly lethal diagnosis had been confirmed. And although his survival to this point was already considered extraordinary, there was no way to know what lay ahead.

Slowly he began to tell his story:

I am not a sickly person. In thirty-two years, I had never missed more than one day of work down at the plant. No one there knew I wasn't up to par except the fellow I worked with every day. For thirty-two years, I worked nine hours a day, six days a week at the mill.

It started with a pain between my shoulder blades. It was real strong pain. I went to the doctor immediately. He did a complete physical and then sent me home again.

I could stand it during the day, but I couldn't stand it at night. It was getting worse every day.

You can't sleep with pain like that. I tried sleeping in the bathtub in hot water. I forget all the things I tried to sleep, but you can't sleep with pain like that.

I kept working nine hours a day at the mill. The day I left, that was it—I never went back.

It got to be Thursday, and the doctor couldn't find anything on me. I called him back and asked what he was doing. He said, "I'll put you in the hospital on Monday." I told him, "No, you're not, you're going to put me in today or else I'm going down myself." So he says, "I'll put you in the hospital tonight." That was August 20, 1981. All they did at Johnson was dope me. (He turns to Lillian.) How long was I in Johnson Hospital?

[Lillian answered his questions and soon was adding details to Walter's account.]

Lillian: Walter was in Johnson over a weekend. A weekend isn't a good time to be in a hospital. Then on the following Tuesday he was transferred to Mercy Hospital. Once he got down there, they started the tests, and things moved quickly. All this time, the pain was still intense. He couldn't lie down. He sat in a chair or moved around. On Friday, they had it all diagnosed, what was wrong with him.

Walter: I had no idea I had cancer. They finally tapped my spine, and that's where they found the cancer. In the liquid in the spine, I guess it's liquid, I don't know.

L: I can't remember word for word what the doctor said to me, but it was horrible. He said that Walter should get his affairs in order. They said that he could have treatments or not have any treatments. They didn't think anything would do any good.

W: They told me what it was. They told everybody else, too. I never did think I was going to die. Never did.

L: They didn't think treatments would do Walter any good really.

W: I never had the feeling I would die. I probably should have. I knew that it was serious, but I didn't realize then how much time I was supposed to have.

L: It's hard to tell what caused it. The doctors wanted to know if he worked with chemicals. They have asbestos in the mill, like any of these old buildings. They have since taken it down. It's hard to tell. It's not like he's a smoker.

W: Well, Lillian always said I ate too many sweets. From everything I hear, I gather that's about the worst thing you can eat.

L: The doctor told me what was available. Then we, Walter and I, decided. We knew people who had radiation and then became terribly ill from it, so we decided that we didn't want any part of it. But Walter was having so much trouble with his eyes; he couldn't see well. He was having trouble with his whole face. So when it came right down to it, we decided that we would have it, that maybe the treatment would help.

W: We certainly wanted something, even though there wasn't any possible chance. We wanted to survive as long as possible. They transferred me over to...

L: Bayside Medical Center. You had your first treatment on Saturday.

W: Normally they don't give any treatments on Saturday. But I told them I wanted it, so they brought a nurse in specially for that.

L: [Lillian looked at Walter.] You were so determined. Even though it seemed hopeless, he'd still go through the motions of doing different things. For whatever reason, he was very determined. To me, the doctor's always right. That's the difference between us, I guess. When the doctor said "This is it," to me that was it. But Walter wasn't going to take that for nothing.

W: At first, they gave me an old room, and I don't know who did it, Lillian or my brother, but they got me out of that old room and put me in a new one.

I was having an awful lot of hallucinations at night from the painkillers. Then the next night I'd go right on with the same hallucination. But I never stopped using the bathroom, walking around. That was against my wife's wishes.

L: He's plain stubborn, always has been.

W: I had the piles, and this one nurse did an awfully rough job of flushing me out. He was a male nurse, and he, of course, had to give me the enema. After he gave me the enema, I had a bad case of... what was it I had?

L: Hemorrhoids.

W: Hemorrhoids. That really hurt. I had a nurse that hurt me every time she gave me the medicine for that. All the rest of the nurses didn't. So I finally spoke to her, and she straightened out. But I had excellent care while I was in the hospital.

I had good company, too. I was in with this other fella that had heart trouble. He wasn't supposed to smoke. One day he lit up a cigarette just as his wife comes in the door. She looked. She turned around and never came back. [Walter and Lillian laughed.] That was a little strange, but she didn't want him to smoke.

L: He got wonderful care, wonderful care. I couldn't complain at all; they're very caring at Baystate and Mercy.

He did have tremendous support from everybody. All our friends and family would go to see him. There were prayers from California, and Maine, Vermont, and New Hampshire, from all over the country, and that helped a lot. Our friends and family would ask people in other churches to pray. All that love helped Walter get better.

W: Must've been something like that. Many of 'em prayed right here, right at the house. It seems that helped. Even up to Alaska, they prayed up at the church where Uncle Julius goes.

I got a box of get-well cards in there that's this high and this wide [about two feet by three feet]. Here, let me show you. Someday I'm going to read them all again.

L: You had a great deal of comforting. One day the whole room was filled with people. There were fourteen people in his room.

W: Mostly relatives. My brother came up from Georgia. I had more visitors than anybody, didn't I?

L: Yes.

W: It seemed that way, anyway.

L: When he left Baystate, they hadn't made arrangements for him to have a treatment that day. But he insisted on having a treatment that day. It was too late to do it there, so they called Cooley Dickinson Hospital, and he got it on the way home.

W: They cancelled my treatment for the day. I can't believe they would pull a stunt like that. So I got after them and told them how I wanted the treatment before I went home. When I was discharged, I went down every other day for treatment.

L: He had twenty-two in all. Fourteen on his head, because he had an outbreak of it at the base of his skull. He had the maximum amount allowed. He can't ever have any more. After the treatment, his doctor said Walter hadn't responded.

W: My doctor said the radiation didn't do any good. But I wouldn't have wanted to try without it.

I felt a lot of pain when I finished the radiation.

See my face? Everything just drooped right down. Like this! My eyes went dry. This was after I got home. They caused me an awful lot of pain. They wouldn't work. I couldn't shut them. I was in tough shape for a while.

L: His eyelids wouldn't close. They'd dry out. At night, we had to tape them shut.

W: My doctor had just made contact with an acupuncturer. He came up to see if he could drum up a little business, and I, of course, was the logical patient. Dr. Lesser asked if I was interested. It's nothing I would have thought of, but he wanted to get me off the heavy dosage of Demerol. I agreed.

All of this was brand-new. All new. We were open because I knew I needed healing. I went there fifty-two times.

My eyes were way down here [Walter held his hand a few inches in front of his eyes] when I started going over. It seemed to make me better.

He gave me the needles. He used to say, "Take a deep breath," and then you blow out and then bang, he zips it right in. But after a while I got so I didn't have to do that anymore. I just says, "Knock 'em in wherever you want." I remember he stuck one right up under my upper lip. I said, "That one hurt worse than anything. I don't think you did it right." The next time, he pushed it in all at once instead of tapping it four times.

The acupuncture was very important though I don't think it chased the illness out.

We highly recommend him, but not everybody would like him. We do. I do.

L: What do you mean, "Not everyone would like him?" You mean not like the treatment 'cause John is such a nice person, I'm sure everybody would like him. I think it helped, too, to talk with him while Walter was having the treatment. He's very quiet, a very nice person.

Another interesting thing: Walter went to an eye, nose, throat specialist in Springfield. He was given tests, and the doctor said that, on this really fine instrument to measure nerve conduction, there was no response. Walt hadn't been to John for more than three weeks of acupuncture when he started to move his facial muscles. He really came along quite fast.

W: He charged us only ten dollars for two hours. Amazing. I think he charges more for other people.

L: He should. That's too little, to spend two hours with a person for ten dollars.

W: The pain kept getting less and less, so I finally did stop going.

I called him up a while ago, and I told him I was coming down just to visit. But he likes to stick needles in ya, so if you go visit him you'll be laying on his table with needles comin' out of ya. It feels good.

And the acupuncturer took me to the Tibetan doctor. What's his name?

L: Dr. Dhonden.*

W: We liked him. He would take a tube of urine and almost tell you what was the matter with ya just by looking at that. He was a good doctor.

L: He told John [the acupuncturist] that he could cure Walter in two years. And Walter took the medicine faithfully until he ran out, and we couldn't get any more. Well, maybe that cured it, who knows?

W: He told me that sweets were about the worst thing I could eat. So now, I eat practically no sweets. I don't have any liquor. I used to drink occasionally, not steady, just when we'd go out on Saturday nights. And no coffee at all. That's about it.

He was a good doctor. I was taking these pills, they're herbs, for quite a while. He says they can get rid of the cancer, whereas the people from here say they can't. You know, if he hadn't had any faith, I don't believe that I would have.

And I went to my cousin's wife who treats people with the concentration of her hands.

She just holds her hands right over your body, especially where you're sick. You can almost feel it, the transfer of—not heat—it's a transfer of energy. It's hard to believe, but it seems you could feel it. She showed Lillian how to do it. Lillian did it quite a few times. She didn't seem to have quite as much enthusiasm about it as this girl had. She was really for it. She teaches it.

Lillian didn't care if I got those treatments or not, but I kept after her to give them to me.

I never felt like throwing in the towel. Maybe you did, Lillian, but I didn't.

L: No, you didn't.

W: You asked why I did better than most people with the illness. Well, things don't bother me too much. I just don't let things worry me at all. I always had a pretty easy temperament. I didn't yell and scream at people. I still don't. I didn't get discouraged. I never thought I wasn't going to get better. Maybe that's the reason,

*At the time of the interview, Dr. Yeshi Dhonden was the personal physician for the Dalai Lama.

because I'm easygoing. I have a friend who bought me a tape that I use quite a bit, and I'll let you listen to it. It's called... Lillian, what's it called?

L: Meditation.

W: Meditation, that's it. I can't remember too good. I think when they put the radiation through my head, they took part of the brains out. [Walter laughed.] I don't worry about that either.

[Walter took me into the bedroom, where a tape recorder rested on a chair next to his bed. The recording he wanted me to hear was a Simonton Relaxation Tape. The portion I listened to instructs the listener to systematically relax different parts of the body.]

I listen to it twice a day. It relaxes your whole body.

L: A neighbor just came down with cancer. Walter brought it over to her right away.

W: I sure relax more than before. I'm a great TV fan, and I usually spend each morning watching TV. In the afternoon, I get out and do something outdoors. I move around everyday.

Take a look at that cuckoo clock. I started fixing clocks as soon as I got home from the hospital. I enjoy doing that. Here's an antique grandfather clock that I've been working on since I got sick. I can make it talk, but I can't make it run. I stopped working on it when the weather got good. Now I should be finishing it up shortly.

I have a good time—as long as I don't get worse. I enjoy what I'm doing now. I didn't enjoy what I was doing before.

I can do so many of the things now that I never had time for before, working six days a week, nine hours a day.

I have a pretty good amount of energy; but if I stay up too late, then I get worn down quicker. I can do a lot of things, but not everything. I tried to help a neighbor in putting a roof on up. But I just couldn't squat down to work on the roof.

[A very powerful moment of the interview came when I asked Walter, "While you were so ill, why did you want to live? What were the reasons—" Walter interrupted me, the only time he did in all the hours we spent together:]

I wasn't that sick. Oh, I was real sick, but I never lost the will to get better. I appreciate everything we do much more. A couple months back, I went up to Alaska on a fishing trip. My brother, my son, and

I went salmon fishing, red salmon. I could walk right up the side of the brook; it was uphill for two miles, and I could keep right up with the rest of them. I don't know where all the energy came from. We had a wonderful time.

[To close the interview, I asked Walter to summarize why he thought he was so much more successful than expected.]
Everything helped. That's for sure. But I swear we never knew for sure.

About six months after meeting with the Puringtons, while I was speaking with a group of hospice volunteers, I met, by chance, a volunteer who had worked with Walter. This elderly man told me that even while Walter was so sick, he used to describe all the activities he planned to do, such as fishing in Alaska and learning to snowmobile. The volunteer said that at the time he assumed, like everyone else familiar with the case, that Walter was simply denying the seriousness of his condition.

Walter later became the first person ever to be discharged alive from this hospice program. When the volunteer's wife was hospitalized following a heart attack, the roles of helper and helpee were reversed as Walter drove the man to the hospital, offering comfort and support.

In the second interview, we covered much of the same ground as in the first one. But the feel was entirely different. Five years had passed, and the cancer was no longer an ever-present threat. The tension I experienced during the first interview, fearful that I might do something "wrong," was gone. I felt free to enjoy Walter's remarkable story and the Purington Yankee warmth.

Walter was not big on words, but the covert communication was loud and clear. Before the interview even began, Walter let me know that he was eager to help me learn everything I could about him and his experience. Within minutes of this return visit, he said that there was something I should see. He led me downstairs for a tour of the cellar. He showed me the beer his son-in-law was distilling, the herb garden his wife was growing, and the woodburner he had installed to heat their home.

One facet of Walter's beauty was his concreteness. He literally demonstrated his willingness to share whatever was in his head. Back at the kitchen table, he pulled a Q-tip out of its box and explained that his ears have caused him trouble since the radiation treatment. He proudly showed me his own personal technique for lubricating and cleaning his ears. The technique, he said, was superior to the one shown to him by a specialist. As if for proof, he produced a chunk of wax for me to examine.

Walter showed the same willingness to share his innermost thoughts. Access, however, was more of a problem as his tendency to act rather than reflect seemed to increase with his growing good health.

I wondered if his children had moved out of the house since we last met. He instructed me to look out the window on my left. About 300 yards away was a small white Cape Cod house. "My daughter and her husband built that one."

"Now go look out that window," he said, pointing to the one on my right. Perched on the top of the closest hill was another house. "That's my other daughter's. Moved back from New York after I got sick."

Walter continued, "The mules, did you see some mules on the road when you forked right? Well, those belong to my son and his wife. They live just down the road a piece. He's moving to Maine—must know I'm OK now."

Walter said that he was still eating as he had five years before—a balanced diet with little alcohol. He was eating more sweets, but nothing like before the cancer: "I hardly ever have more than one chocolate bar at a time now."

He took me all around the house and grounds, sharing pieces of his life with me. He showed me a couple of snowmobiles he and Lillian had purchased last year. He seemed surprised when I asked if he went out on them. In his mind, apparently, there was only one reason why he wouldn't take part in this strenuous winter play: "Well, the snow's been bad this year, but we're hoping for more."

Walter then let me know that his improving health had not been a steady upward climb.

You pretty near missed me. I was getting darn low. When they gave me radiation, it went right to my head. Knocked out the pituitary gland. Knocked it right out. And from that day, my body went down, steady downhill for five years. If you come here a year quicker, you'd have found me pretty near crawling. I wasn't crawling, but the doctor said I should have been. My pituitary wasn't feeding my thyroid.

I got up one morning and couldn't talk. Just a garble. I went to the couch and laid down. Two girls come in I hadn't seen for a couple of years, I perked right up when they came in, but I knew I was in trouble.

I called up and made an appointment with Dr. Morrow. He checked me out all the way from the top of my head to my toes. It took him about an hour to do each side. He started checking my neck. He never found the thyroid. Everything else was running good. As a last resort, he shipped me out to Dr. Shaw.

[Lillian joined in the conversation:]
That was just last spring. Dr. Shaw said he was amazed that Walter could walk into his office with the condition of his thyroid. Apparently there was some hormone there for a while, but it just kept producing less and less; therefore, he was going down. The oncologists were looking for more cancer, but that wasn't it. Dr. Shaw spotted the problem right off. He was so sure it was his thyroid that he started him on thyroid medication even before he got the blood test back. Since the summer, there has been a big improvement.

W: After they found out about the thyroid, that it had stopped working from the radiation, Lillian and I climbed Mount Monadnock. We didn't go to the top, but we came awful close.

Just for the fun of it, would you be interested in seeing what I have to take every day? [Walter went to one of the nearby cabinets and pulled down four bottles. He then showed me the five pills he took every day.] I'm not a pill man, you know. I never knew how to take pills before. I take all of these at once, and they tell me to throw in an aspirin. It's to keep your heart from kicking you over some night.

Several of my old buddies have dropped out this year. Everyone thought I'd be the first to drop out.

When I went back to Dr. Case, he said that the whole hospital staff had a meeting on my particular case. He said they just couldn't figure out how they made a mistake. He said they went through all the records, and they came up with the same conclusion: that I couldn't pull through it. So they sent the prints, the slides, the X-rays, and everything to Duke University. They came up with the same diagnosis that the hospital did; they said that I couldn't pull through it. I didn't know that until after I started to get pretty good.

[At the end of the interview, I asked the same question I had asked five years before, "Why do you think you did so well?" Walter answered:]

I never gave up. I didn't want to die; I still don't. Even today I feel that I have quite a few more years, good years, left.

L: It's true. His frame of mind is probably a big reason. He never appeared to have gotten depressed, he was just always plugging along.

W: I'd like to try the whole thing again—only this time have them catch the thyroid problem quicker.

OBSERVATIONS

At first glance, the facts and figures suggest that Walter was an unlikely candidate to try alternative therapies. For thirty years, he had worked in the same job, at the same mill. He had lived in the same small rural town for fifty years, married to the same woman for twenty-eight years. His previous exposure to medical treatment of any kind was extremely limited and always traditional. How then are we to understand his openness to approaches that ran the gamut from traditional to exotic?

Exploring Walter's personality and the situation in which he found himself is one way to begin. Lillian states, and Walter provides verification, that persistence and determination were his core characteristics. When he became ill, this determination was entirely focused toward health. There was no ambivalence draining his life energies: He was willing to do whatever it took to get well.

His inexperience with illness may have served him well. Since Walter was a beginner he was not limited by his preconceptions about the way one recovers from serious illness. Unlike his oncologists, who were bound by their repertoire of chemotherapy, radiation, and surgery, Walter never lost hope or felt that there were no other avenues to pursue. Since Walter was never dependent upon traditional medical practice, the physicians' announcement that they had no answers was not a death verdict. He still believed that they had something valuable to offer. Indeed he had more faith in the value of their methods than they did and so insisted on radiation. But there was no reason to totally rely on a system that explicitly said the health he so desired was beyond its power to achieve.

Knowing that he "needed some healing," Walter set off to find it. He was much too ill, however, to journey far or to actively seek out options. Instead his determination took the form of opening to possibilities as they arose. Thus, when his family doctor suggested acupuncture, he went for fifty-two treatments. When his acupuncturist told him about a famed Tibetan doctor, Walter traveled considerable distances to meet with Yeshi Dhonden and then faithfully followed a regimen of herbs and diet change. When he learned that a relative healed through a laying on of hands or when a neighbor mentioned the Simonton stress relaxation exercises, he tried them with enthusiasm and commitment, believing that they could help to heal him.

For someone so ill, Walter remained remarkably potent in all aspects of his treatment. After a nurse treated him in a disrespectful manner, he did what was necessary to change this person's behavior. When Walter felt the acupuncturist had misdirected a needle, he did not hesitate to tell him so. And when normal bureaucratic procedures dictated that he would not receive treatment on the day of discharge, he demanded the treatment and received it.

Obviously Walter would do whatever he could to influence the course of his illness. But it was really the combination of his strong will and acceptance that made him such an interesting and rare individual. He did battle with cancer like Krishna in the *Bhagavad Gita*, who said: "Prepare for war with peace in Thy soul." He was a peaceful warrior, ever vigilant to threats and opportunities, yet accepting of his human limitations. Knowing that he had done everything possible in his quest for health, he could accept any outcome. We saw a remarkable example of this in the interview. After fumbling unsuccessfully for the third time to retrieve a word, Walter commented that the radiation had knocked out part of his brain; but, instead of being upset by such a major loss, he commented, ''I don't worry about that either.''

Only in context can we fully appreciate Walter's ability to stay centered while maintaining his desire to stay alive. Walter was not just dealing with the emotional aspects of a terminal prognosis. The physical pain and discomfort was extreme. In *No Exit*, by Jean Paul Sartre, three characters suddenly find themselves together with no understanding of where they are or how they got there. As the story progresses, we suspect that they are in hell. Learning that they have no eyelids, so even a moment of respite is impossible, our suspicions are confirmed.

Walter's condition resembled a similar kind of hell. The pain was intense, and he could not close his eyelids without assistance. The idea that illness is in part subjective is poignantly demonstrated by his answer to the question ''Why did you want to get better?'' When he responded, ''I wasn't that sick,'' we know that his reality was very different from the reality others perceived.

According to Walter, the loving care he received from Lillian and the community, but especially from Lillian, contributed to his healing. Lillian's participation in the interview, though I had not specifically asked her to take part, reflected her total involvement in all phases of the disease and treatment. In fact, Lillian was so connected with Walter that she did not feel that he alone was receiving the treatment. As Lillian said, ''When it came right down to it, *we* decided that *we* would have it, that maybe the treatment would help.'' Walter communicated a parallel sentiment. Together they were an entity—a couple with a distinct and precious existence of its own. ''*We* certainly wanted something even though there wasn't any possible chance. *We* wanted to survive as long as possible.'' Sustaining the relationship was an important reason to stay alive.

Walter's competitive spirit may have been subtle, but it was constant, strong, and deep. He compared himself to others to see how he measured up. The fact that he had ''more visitors than anybody'' confirmed that people cared about and valued him. He was proud that he was not the first one in their circle of friends to ''drop out,'' despite his deadly disease. His competitive nature gave him another reason to keep going while so ill and to achieve what others before him had not been able to.

Some of the support Walter found in the environment may have simply been the result of circumstance or good fortune. But it is important to recognize that Walter was responsible for creating the milieu he needed. For example, there was practically no one, besides himself, who believed that survival was possible. Without someone else to share and nurture this faith, eventual despair seemed inevitable. He found a wellspring of hope in Dr. Dhonden. As Walter told us, "If he hadn't had any faith, I don't believe that I would have."

Despite Walter's New England provincialism, his encounter with Eastern medical healers was more familiar than foreign in significant ways. Shared values provided the common ground. Walter, a man who could be identified as an old Yankee, was honest and forthright with himself as well as others. His basic philosophical stance was "Any job worth doing is worth doing right," whether it was some mundane task or the job of living. We experienced his desire for perfection, however elusive such a goal always is, when he made the remarkable statement, "I'd like to try the whole thing again—only this time . . ."

Yeshi Dhonden's way of life may be more ceremonial and conscious than Walter's, but the two men share a commitment to quality, a commitment to life itself. In *Mortal Lessons*, Richard Selzer, M.D., describes the way Yeshi Dhonden practices medicine:

> On the bulletin board in the front hall of the hospital where I work, there appeared an announcement. "Yeshi Dhonden," it read, "will make rounds at six o'clock on the morning June 10." . . . I am not so leathery a skeptic that I would knowingly ignore an emissary from the gods. Not only might such sangfroid be inimical to one's earthly well-being, it could take care of eternity as well. Thus on the morning of June 10, I join the clutch of whitecoats waiting in the small conference room adjacent to the ward selected for the rounds. The air in the room is heavy with ill-concealed dubiety and suspicion of bamboozlement. At precisely six o'clock he materializes, a short, golden, barrelly man dressed in a sleeveless robe of saffron and maroon. His scalp is shaven, and the only visible hair is a scanty black line above each hooded eye.
>
> He bows in greeting while his young interpreter makes the introduction. Yeshi Dhonden, we are told, will examine a patient selected by a member of the staff. The diagnosis is unknown to Yeshi Dhonden as it is to us. . . . We are further

informed that for the past two hours Yeshi Dhonden has purified himself by bathing, fasting, and prayer. . . .

Yeshi Dhonden steps to the bedside while the rest stand apart, watching. For a long time he gazes at a woman. . . . I, too, study her. No physical sign or obvious symptom gives a clue to the nature of her disease.

At last he takes her hand, raising it in both of his own. Now he bends over the bed in a kind of crouching stance, his head drawn down into the collar of his robe. His eyes are closed as he feels for her pulse. In a moment he has found the spot, and for the next half-hour he remains thus, suspended above the patient like some exotic golden bird with folded wings, holding the pulse of the woman beneath his fingers, cradling her hand in his. All the power of the man seems to have been drawn down to this one purpose. It is palpation of the pulse raised to the state of ritual. . . . I cannot see their hands joined in a correspondence that is exclusive, intimate, his fingertips receiving the voice of her sick body through the rhythm and throb she offers at her wrist. All at once I am envious—not of him, not of Yeshi Dhonden for his gift of beauty and holiness, but of her. I want to be held like that, touched so, *received*. And I know that I, who have palpated a hundred thousand pulses, have not felt a single one.

At last Yeshi Dhonden straightens, gently places the woman's hand upon the bed, and steps back. The interpreter produces a small wooden bowl and two sticks. Yeshi Dhonden pours a portion of the urine specimen into the bowl and proceeds to whip the liquid with two sticks. This he does for several minutes until a foam is raised. Then, bowing above the bowl, he inhales the odor three times. He sets down the bowl and turns to leave. All this while, he has not uttered a single word. . . . "Thank you, doctor," she says, and touches with her other hand the place he had held on her wrist, as though to recapture something that had visited there. . . .

We are seated once more in the conference room. Yeshi Dhonden speaks now for the first time. . . . He speaks of winds coursing through the body of the woman, currents that break against barriers, eddying. These vortices are in her blood, he says. The last spendings of an imperfect heart.

Between the chambers of the heart, long, long before she was born, a wind had come and blown open a deep gate that must never be opened. Through it charge the full waters of her river, as the mountain stream cascades in the springtime, battering, knocking loose the land, and flooding her breath. Thus he speaks, and now he is silent.

"May we now have the diagnosis?" a professor asks.

The host of these rounds, the man who knows, answers.

"Congenital heart disease," he says. "Interventricular septal defect, with resultant heart failure."

A gateway in the heart, I think. That must not be opened. Through it charge the full waters that flood her breath. So! Here then is the doctor listening to the sounds of the body to which the rest of us are deaf. He is more than doctor. He is priest.

I know...I know...the doctor to the gods is pure knowledge, pure healing. . . .

Now and then it happens, as I make my own rounds, that I hear the sounds of his voice, like an ancient Buddhist prayer, its meaning long since forgotten, only the music remaining. Then a jubilation possesses me, and I feel myself touched by something divine.

RELATED RESEARCH

Despite the message of hopelessness, Walter never thought he would succumb to the illness. There are many studies that indirectly point to a relationship between hope and survival. One study placed rats in situations that were either hopeful or hopeless. Though the sadism of the researcher is an open question, the findings are relevant. After rats were put in water, the experimenter watched to see how long it would take them to die. Death was due to electrical abnormalities (roughly equivalent to a heart attack or seizure) and not drowning. The rats that were held tightly in the experimenter's hand—leaving no hope for survival—died the quickest.

Generally, wild rats died from one to fifteen minutes after immersion in the water. However, the researcher found that if rats were placed in the water and then repeatedly rescued, they survived much longer—up to eighty-one hours. It can be hypothesized that these rats "knew" that there was hope and consequently did not give up.

The functioning of Walter's immune system was probably enhanced by his ability to respond peacefully to even the most traumatic of life events. While research cannot yet conclude that a definitive relationship exists between human cancer growth and stress,* it appears close. For many years, a host of studies have demonstrated that stressors of various types could weaken the functioning of the immune system. At the Ohio State University School of Medicine, researchers found that a stressor (academic exams) could suppress the body's ability to produce natural killer cells—lymphoid immune cells that help prevent the development of tumors. And Drs. Alfred Amkraut and George Solomon discovered that after mice were inoculated with a virus to induce tumors, the tumors of stressed mice (they were given electric shocks) grew faster than the tumors of unstressed mice.

In another study, researchers actually predicted which people in a sample would develop cancer. Fifty-one women whose pap tests demonstrated atypical cervical cytology ("suspicious cells" indicating a high probability of developing cancer) were interviewed and given a battery of psychological tests. Drs. Arthur Schmale and Howard Iker hypothesized that the women who seemed to feel helpless and hopeless would develop cancer; the rest would not. Using only this criterion, their predictions of malignancy were correct 73.6 percent of the time.

Any attempt to measure the effect of a loving relationship like the one enjoyed by Walter and Lillian would be interesting but necessarily simplistic. Research does seem to indicate, however, that married individuals fare better with their cancer than single people. A study published by the *Journal of the American Medical Association* (1987) used data on 27,779 cancer cases from the New Mexico Tumor Registry. They found that married people have a 23 percent higher survival rate than single individuals. Dr. Walter Goodwin, the lead researcher, said that married people are likely to get diagnosed earlier, and early diagnosis improves probability of survival. Even after this factor is

---

*Our use of the term stress suggests dis-stress or dis-ease, a nonfunctional response that is maladaptive to the situation. It is not simply referring to the dynamic tension that results from the distance between one's present state and desired state.

discounted, however, married people are still more likely to survive their cancer. He said, "For that we have no explanation," but speculated that the emotional support they received from their spouses could account for the difference. Clearly, Lillian gave emotional support to Walter, but just as important was the meaning that their marital relationship brought into his life. It gave him reason to stay alive.

KURT METZLER

If you want to know how it feels, take in a deep breath, let it half way out, now try and take in a deep breath again. That's how it feels all the time. For me, that's normal.

Kurt Metzler

A friend of mine, who has a brown belt in karate, first told me about Kurt Metzler. She said that about seven years ago, a young man showed up for a karate class. This man did not attend class nearly so often as other serious students, but his capacity to focus on the training and his understanding of his body's capabilities and limitations set him apart from all the others. Because of his frequent coughing and extended absences, my friend suspected he might be suffering from an illness, yet his ability to perform suggested otherwise. She was surprised to learn from another student that Kurt had cystic fibrosis and would probably be dead within a few years.

Since Kurt was about five years old, people have been assuming that he would die shortly. During our interviews, Kurt offered many examples of this. The most recent: "Last month, I went to a high school reunion. My old classmates were very surprised to see me. I didn't know this because no one talked to me about it, but the word around school was that I wouldn't live past twenty. Everyone was expecting me to croak anytime soon."

The anticipation of his death was then and is now based on statistics. The specialist most familiar with Kurt's course of illness said that the probability he could survive to the age of thirty was 1 in 1,000. Kurt is thirty-one. A second physician, who corroborated the extraordinary nature of his continued survival, was asked why he thought Kurt did so well. He speculated, "Good luck?"

Before meeting with Kurt, my knowledge of cystic fibrosis was limited. But from what I did know about the ravages of the disease, it seemed safe to assume that he would appear sickly.

When I arrived at his home, Kurt opened the door, shook my hand, then reached out to take my bag filled with recording equipment. He looked like an athlete. His handshake was firm, and even while carrying my heavy bag he maintained the spring in his step. He was bowlegged, but the curvature did not look like the crippling effects of an illness but rather the mark of a football player or weightlifter whose body had adapted over time to provide maximum stability and strength. It may seem odd, but it was not until the interview began and Kurt was describing the illness and its effects on his body that I realized he was five feet one and not quite 110 pounds.

He was cute, not in an impish sort of way, but the kind of cute that came from feeling confident enough to give free rein to his playfulness. His huge smile opened his face, and he was sure enough of his own masculinity that he could allow others to glimpse his vulnerability. I felt awed by the grueling physical and emotional pace that Kurt kept up day after day.

The interviews were conducted at his parents home in Greenfield, Massachusetts. Kurt has an apartment in the same town but was housesitting for the winter. He explained, "My parents went camping cross-country. They're getting older, and they've decided to do the things they've always wanted to do while they still can." He thought for a minute and said with a laugh, "I guess that's really what I'm doing." The story he tells reveals just how true these words are:

I'm obsessed. Some people are obsessed with money, others are obsessed with success, others with fame, and so they direct all their energy toward that particular goal. I'm obsessed with being well. I have to be. I got the drive from my parents; they gave me the good start. My father is an obsessive worker. He made the clock there, the furniture we're sitting on; he makes violins. He wired the house himself; he's a carpenter, a welder. He does everything well. He has a drive that I envy; I think, growing up, we all did. If I had been healthy, I would have been just like him—able to do the same things. But because of the disease, I put all of my energies into fighting an illness and staying healthy.

Sometimes after work people are going out and they'll ask me, "Do you want to come?" I want to go, to meet with friends, to talk, to relax and laugh. But I know I can't—that's the hardest part. I have to do what I have to do. I have to go home and pound on myself.

I do therapy twice a day. I lie on a board upside down and pound the chest to get some of the stuff out of my lungs. I can do everything myself except for the back. I have a machine, a compressor, hooked to a vibrator—sounds a little sexy—a percussion type of instrument that I hold to my back. It helps.

When I was born, the average life expectancy for someone with cystic fibrosis was eight years. I'm thirty-one years old now. Obviously, the doctors were wrong in my case.

Every day, I have to get out and exercise. I go out and run every night; if it's real cold I'll run inside, but I have to do it every day. Jogging is basic. Now I jog about a mile a day. I used to jog four miles. But the lungs decided that they didn't like that, and they were hemorrhaging. If I stop doing this, if I stopped exercising, I probably wouldn't be around in four months.

It's a balancing act. Too much exercise will be damaging, and not enough will be damaging. So I'm constantly juggling.

I've seen a lot of people with CF over the years who didn't have the drive to constantly stay at it, and they're not around anymore. There used to be five people from this area who would go to the clinic. The last one died about eight or nine years ago. Seeing them, seeing that they weren't doing as well as I was, would drive home the point not to end up like them.

I've known one other person who also did very, very well. When I was younger, I used to go to this clinic with . . . Oh, God, I forgot his name . . . Rossberg. We went together every couple of months, so we became fairly close. He was a few years older than I was. He got me into exercising, into weightlifting, when I was in junior high. He did well.

I went to see him in the hospital about four or five days before he died. He didn't look too bad. As we were walking out, my mom says, "You know, he's dying."

I said, "What?"

"He's dying. He isn't going to make it. The doctor says maybe a week." I was shocked then, but after he died I said, "Well, it only goes to show you: If you stop, you're going to pay for it."

When he went away to college in Hawaii, he stopped the therapy, the exercising. I don't know why. I bet he would still be here today if he hadn't stopped.

I think his death may have helped me. It was proof, and it may have given me a little more drive to keep the routine going.

There were differences between Rossberg and me. I was always more tied to home—he was more on his own. I think I had a stronger home base. My family has been very important. They can't keep me healthy, but they have a big influence.

Cystic fibrosis is a problem with the lungs and the pancreas. The lungs secrete a mucus. With a normal person, it'll be a thin mucus that gets dirt and other junk out. In the case of a cystic fibrosis patient, the mucus is a lot thicker and a lot heavier. It does not come out, so it will sit there, become infected, and it becomes a breeding ground for infection. I've been hospitalized, I bet, fifteen, sixteen, maybe even twenty times. They bring me into the hospital for ten days to two weeks, and they pump antibiotics into me—intravenously, because that's the best way to get to the infection. With pills, the stomach tends to destroy the effects of the antibiotics.

But the infection scars the lungs. Eventually the alveoli, which are really tiny air sacs, get scarred and grow together. Since this decreases the surface area, your lung capacity drops. I can breathe in 1.8 liters in one deep breath, whereas a normal person can do something like four quarts. My illness, then, is quite severe. Eventually, the lungs cannot function anymore and the patient dies.

And the problems aren't just with the lungs. The pancreas does not secrete enough enzymes to digest food. So everything passes right through you without your body pulling the nutrients out. CF patients don't grow up to full size because they're chronically undernourished. I'm sure if I was normal, I'd be bigger. To help with digestion, I take enzymes.

Some people have just digestive problems, others just lung problems. Some people have both lung and digestive problems, but they have it mildly. I happen to have both severely. Yet I think I'm in the best shape of anyone I've seen with CF. I think through exercise my body has learned to use what it has available to maximum efficiency.

I've decided to do the things I want while I still can. Like, many years ago, I went with a church group to climb Mount Washington. We got up halfway and the weather was bad. I decided it was better not to try. So I went back down with another person.

A few years ago, I said, "I tried once and I failed. I want to do it." This time I went with just the minister; he's a friend, even though I don't go to church much. We started up on a Saturday morning. I was stopping a lot. We got up to Tuckerman's Ravine, and black clouds were billowing overhead; it looked really bad. For the last thousand yards or so, we had to climb over these big boulders. It was windy—70 miles an hour, and the temperature was only 40 degrees, even though it was the middle of July. I was experiencing a lack of oxygen, and my legs were cramping up—the whole bowl of wax. I was exhausted. Finally we made it to the top. I don't think I could ever do it again. It took everything out of me, but I'm glad I did it.

When we got there, it was kind of funny because this woman comes over to me from her car. There's also an access road to the top of the mountain. I'm in my hiking shorts, hiking boots, rain gear, walking stick, bent over trying to catch my breath. She says, "Did you really climb all the way up!?" I thought, "No shit, lady."

Last winter, I said to my minister friend, "Why don't we go up again, climb up to Tuckerman's, and I'll ski down?" That means hauling your skis up on your back. We were all set to go. But the day we were scheduled to leave, it was raining, so we had to cancel.

Who knows, I may get there yet.

My goal is to slow down the progress of the illness as much as possible. That's all I can do. It will get worse. It has gotten worse. There's a difference between the way I feel now and the way I felt two or three years ago. On tests it doesn't show up dramatically, but physically I can tell.

When I jogged ten years ago, the adrenaline was really flowing. There was much more of a rush when I was finished. I still get it, but it's nowhere as big. So the lungs are a bit worse off.

I'm still jogging, I'm still pushing it. But when I jog now, I'll feel numbing in my fingers and sometimes a general weakness. I know when I approach the point where I'm not getting enough oxygen and my oxygen levels are beginning to drop. I can tell those subtle differences. Insufficient oxygen levels will cause the heart to work harder. I have to worry about the heart working so hard that it gets damaged.

I did a test at the medical center. They put me on a treadmill and took oxygen levels to see how saturated the blood was with oxygen. After eight minutes of jogging, the oxygen level went down to 60 percent. Anything below that will cause damage if I don't take in more oxygen. From that test, I know how I feel, how the heart feels, right before I reach that critical point. I gauge myself. I push myself that hard but no harder.

Before I went skydiving, I wanted to know if the lack of oxygen could be dangerous. I asked my doctor. He said, "Well, how high are you going?"

I said, "8,000 feet."

"That would be kind of marginal for you."

"Good," I said. "I'll do it." I think the doctor meant it was iffy, iffy. But for me it was a gamble worth taking.

My mother said she wouldn't come to the airfield, but she did for one jump. She noticed that my gums were blue from the altitude, which means I have to watch it.

I'm constantly gauging, if I do this or do that, what will be the effect on me. I was very scared when I first went up, so I had a few people there in case anything happened.

The first time you jump tandem, so it's safer. You're tied to the instructor with two cargo hooks, and you wear a harness attached to him under his belly. You go down like a sandwich, one on top of the other.

I really didn't feel that scared until they opened the plane door. You look out and there's nothing there. You say, "Oh, no." It is cold up there with a strong wind. The first few people go out, and you see them fade away. Phew, OK, so it's your turn, you go out on the side of the plane with your feet hanging out, your rear end right on the edge, and you've got your hand across your chest. The instructor is holding you, and he says, "Ready, ready out we go." You just fall forward and that's it, you're out.

You can do a flip on the way out, and as you come around the plane is leaving. It's sunset, you can look out over the whole horizon. It's such a sensory overload. You can do left turns, right turns, spins, you really have a lot of control. It feels just like you're flying.

Since the pressure up there is a lot less, I can actually breathe easier. I was having such a good time I didn't think about pulling the chute at all. Fortunately the instructor did. The chute opens up and down you float. Next time I go solo.

I saw it on "P.M. Magazine" one night. I said, "I'm going to do that." About a week later, I jumped. I thought, "What the hell! Might as well do it while I still can." I'd always wanted to try.

I'm sure my birth was intense for my parents, but they never talk about it. When I was three hours old, I went in for an eight-hour operation. My intestine was perforated, and there was a blockage.

A few weeks later, when my mother took me home, I was crying a lot, and I wasn't gaining weight. CF babies have foul-smelling bowels. It's disgusting, but that's a sign. My mom knew something was wrong. I went to Dr. Howell in Greenfield. He suspected that I had CF and did a sweat test. They put my hand in the bag, the bag fogged up, and the perspiration was tested. People with CF have a very high salt content in their sweat. That's what he found.

I was born at eight pounds nine ounces. I lost nearly four pounds before my weight stabilized with the enzymes and the low-fat diet.

As a young child, I had to sleep in a mist tent, which I hated. When I was old enough to crawl, I would try to crawl out of it. It would be soaking wet inside the plastic, and who wants to sleep when they're soaking wet? I battled with my parents. I'd sneak out, come downstairs, and go to sleep. I'd be fighting them all the time.

Physical therapy was the worst. I fought them all the way on that one. But they insisted that I stay with it.

I was supposed to take pills, but sometimes I would hide them. When I was five, my father started bribing me, "Take these pills and I'll give you fifty cents. OK?" Ten bucks later, he said, "That's it. I'm cutting you off. No more money." Ever since then, I've been able to take pills by the handfuls.

My own discipline started with the push from my parents. They instilled the idea that I had to exercise, to go out and play, to go running. I know at the time I resented it. I wanted to be a couch potato, but my mother would say, "No, you've got to go out. You have to go play." I used to fight her about it all the time. But together they were relentless as they forced me to keep at it. In retrospect, I realize that they knew better.

They planted the seed that took root. After high school, I took over responsibility for my illness. Now I do have the drive, the presence, the determination to exercise, to do my therapy, to eat right.

It's a good thing, because there are no vacations.

Growing up, I believed that I had done something wrong to make me this way.

My brother or sister were always missing out on this or that because of me—especially family reunions. I'd get sick and I couldn't go, so they couldn't go. It was kind of hard on me, because I felt like I was the cause—and I was. So I constantly felt like I was doing something wrong.

It's ironic, but my sister and brother were jealous of me, jealous of all the attention I got. My sister admitted that at times she hated my guts because so much of my mom's time was spent taking care of me. She hated my guts then, but she and I are closest now.

I got teased a lot when I was in grade school, junior high, and then high school. I was smaller than the other kids. I was only four feet ten, seventy-five pounds when I graduated from high school.

Barrel-chestedness is one effect of the disease. My chest was a little wider than the other kids, and I got teased for that. My teeth were mottled, a side effect of one of the antibiotics, Terramycin. They didn't know then that the tetracyclines can cause permanent discoloration of teeth if taken during tooth development. So I had brown teeth all the way through junior high school and high school. I got teased quite a bit about them, too. Since then, they've been enameled, touched over. But I didn't have it back then.

In school, the pills were embarrassing. At lunch, I would try and sneak all these pills into my hand, like eleven of them, and slug them down at once so the other kids wouldn't know. I became very good at it, but it was a hard secret to keep.

I always thought it was my fault. I never blamed my parents for it. But I think they felt guilty. Mom would express that Dad always felt guilty. CF is genetic. It takes two people with the recessive genes, two people who are carriers. The carriers have no symptoms. They can tell now if someone is a carrier, but back then they couldn't.

Growing up, I always knew that home was safe. We were a close-knit family. It was a very stable environment that I could count on. I was loved.

Many kids with lesser problems got doctor's notes to skip gym. I thought about it, but decided, "Naw, I'll do gym." I would go and do everything all the other kids did. The only problem I had was in basketball, running up and down the court was hard. I tended to fade out. But other than that I did well.

I was a bit of a loner in high school. I could comfortably go from group to group, but I never felt like I really belonged. I joked around a lot and became the class clown. It made me more accepted. I think my insecurity and my pain were the motivation. But being a clown was also natural for me since I've always laughed and joked a lot.

For our school play, we put on *Arsenic and Old Lace*. I played Mutt in the Mutt and Jeff cop team. My partner was two hundred fifty pounds, six feet four. And there I was, only four feet eight, seventy-five pounds. It was a lot of fun.

Another time, in physics class, I had the giggles, and I couldn't stop. My lab partner drew a picture of a cat inside of a dryer, clinging to the sides as it's going around. But I started giggling, and laughing and laughing. I couldn't stop. Everyone was looking at me. The teacher looked at me and said, "Are you through now?" Five minutes later, I started laughing again, but this time the teacher cracked up. Pretty soon the whole class was laughing. I think it's fun to get the giggles; you try and stop and you can't. It leaves a good feeling.

Interesting, though, for me crying has almost the same aftereffect as laughing. But I think I'm all out of crying. In my life, I've done much more laughing. It's easier to laugh. Well, I don't know if it's easier, but you might as well. I mean, why not?

The emotional shit hit the fan when I started college. I got sick. My grades were going downhill. I was feeling, "Where am I going? What can I do with my life? Why should I try and do anything? I'm going to be dead in a couple of years." There were a lot of times when I wished I was dead.

I started seeing a psychologist. I was expecting to have all the answers after one session, to feel better overnight. But it took two or three years before there was much movement.

Therapy made me face some things—like dying. I was having problems with it.

When you're healthy, death seems very far away. Everything is fine. Every time I've gotten sick since I was a little kid, I've had to deal with it, over and over. But I never talked about it.

Many years ago, a doctor advised me not to make any plans more than two years ahead. When he told me that I said, "Fine." But I'm angry about it now. Since I've lived this long, I figure, "Damn, I should have made plans." In fact, doctors have said, "Well, a couple more years and that's it" my whole life. But then it doesn't happen. Sometimes I don't know which way to screw my head on.

All my friends are married with kids, and they're planning their futures. I spend time with them and say, "Uh huh, that's nice." But inside I feel like I'm being left behind.

Therapy helped, but dealing with death isn't simple. It keeps moving. I had begun to feel kind of cocky that finally, after all these years, I had a handle on it. But I don't. I learned that this summer when they were talking transplants. My lungs weren't very healthy then, and I wondered, "Is this it? I really don't want to die. Things are going fairly well." I'll probably be very pissed off when it happens.

The talk about transplants was kind of a shock.

Today, unfortunately, they have to transplant the lungs and heart together. Within the next few years, they'll be transplanting just lungs. The risk of rejection is a lot less when you're playing with only one organ instead of multiple organs.

Of course, heart transplants are a dime a dozen now. And they have done heart and lung transplants. They have transplanted a single lung, but they've only done a few of them. It's a lot more technical to transplant just the lung because you have to reattach it to the heart. That's why it's easier to transplant the lungs and heart together. The doctor says that because I'm young and in a good state of nourishment, as healthy as I can be, I'd be a prime candidate for a transplant. That's what I'm trying to bide time for. I want to keep the damage from the disease to a minimum, waiting it out until technology can catch up to me. The longer I wait, the better the chances.

Once the transplanted lungs are in, there's no more CF. Amazing. No more therapy, no more constant training. I believe I would still do it, but I wouldn't have to. To breathe normally would probably feel like heaven. I can't conceive of it.

But with the transplant, I would be taking on a whole different set of problems. The drugs you take to fight rejection kill all your white blood cells, so you risk infection and colds, kidney problems, stuff like that. But I think the trade-off would be worth it. I'll have a lot more energy; I could do things I can't do now.

I have to figure out when to have the operation. Do I risk it while I'm still relatively healthy? I could be throwing away some good years. Do I wait until I'm on oxygen all the time anyway? But then, since I'd be in a weakened condition, my chances wouldn't be as good. I will talk it over with my parents. I will talk it over with the doctors.

Ultimately the decision will be mine.

Timing is critical, but even once I decide the best time for the operation, there's no guarantee that organs will be available. The stupid part is that I have to apply for and then wait in line for my new organs. When should I do this? I don't want them to come up with a lung all of sudden when I'm too healthy, but I don't want to wait 'til it's too late. It could be months or it could be years before I find one.

I'm trying to hold out as long as I can until they have more experience in the field. The surgery is experimental, techniques are still being developed. I wouldn't want to go through it now. I'm glad I don't have to. I'd rather wait five or ten years down the road.

I'm fearful and careful of colds, of the flu. I know that something small could easily snowball. You never know. Things are going along fine now. If it stays like this, I bet I could go ten, twelve, twenty years. But I'm sure it won't. The disease doesn't stop.

I admit that sometimes I feel depressed. When that happens, I say, "Kurt, knock it off, just do something, walk the dog, go running." It gets my mind off it. If I'm healthy, I get out of it quick, maybe fifteen minutes to an hour. Because I can go do something. It's a lot harder if I'm sick. I realize that, in order to change my mood, I have to do something. Deciding to do something is easy; doing something is the hard part.

I try saying to myself, "Be happy with what you've got. Don't waste time thinking, Oh, if I only had a relationship, or if I only had this or that. It's not worth it. You're just wasting time."

Depressing thoughts about the future come often. But I don't stay with them. Exercise is a good cure for depression. Movement seems to kill the depression.

I do different things. I had a Honda 440, and last year I rode with my friend to Canada on it. A 440 to Canada was kind of ridiculous. You get off the bike, and your hands are still vibrating. It's not like driving a car. All your muscles tense up; it's exhausting. After I got back, I said to heck with that and bought a Kawasaki 650.

I water-ski almost every weekend in the summer. On the Connecticut River, you have to watch out for the dead fish and the tin cans. I'm at the point where I can slalom, get out of the water on one ski, beach-start, stuff like that. I play softball, too, for the company team. In the winter, I roller-skate and ski. Downhill skiing is probably my best sport.

I know it sounds arrogant, but I'm good now. I often wonder how much better I would be if I was normal, if I had the strength, the stamina of a normal person. How good could I be? Because of the physical limitations, I can't go further. That's kind of exasperating.

Moderation is the key. I used to go all out and destroy myself, get sick, stuff like that. But not anymore.

I think I know exactly what the body will take, but sometimes I go over, like in karate. It's hard not to push myself to the limit, especially in testing for a new belt. Testing is much more strenuous than a class. Last December I was tested for my purple belt. At the end, I was so exhausted, I was just lying there, and we still had sparring left. I could feel how drained I was, I was getting a cold because of it. I got up. I was going to fight and lose. I fought, I won. That meant I had to fight again. I said, "Well, I'll lose this time." No, I won again. Well, this kept going. Finally I stopped, but only because the time limit had run out after six hours. I would have gone on. In those situations, if I could just stand up and say, "Kurt, what are you doing? Stop it!" But I don't.

A lot of martial arts teachers are militaristic. But I found a karate teacher, Richard Roy, who tunes in to each individual student. He has an intuitive sense of what will be healing. Twice a day, I do the Chinese breathing exercises he gave me. There's one called "The Tiger Roars": As you inhale, you imagine you're breathing in a cool mist. As you exhale, you push all the air out, and you visualize that the stuff coming out is black and fiery and blaaaak. Once you have completely pushed all the air out, you begin again, by bringing in the cool, clear mist.

Except for the Chinese breathing, I don't do any kind of meditation. It's very difficult for me to sit still. For example, I can't read. Oh, I can read, but I cannot sit down and read for hours at a time, although it might be fun. People seem to get a lot of enjoyment out of books. When I sit, I just see the body filling up. Mentally I start fidgeting, and I can't concentrate. I don't do model building or woodworking or anything that's sedentary. Before we have these conversations, I know that I'll be sitting for longer than usual, so like today, I already went jogging, I cleaned the car, walked the dog. [It was ten A.M. on a Sunday morning]

I've wondered if doctors would ever ask me what I've done to stay so healthy. Obviously not. I think the majority of them are caught up in their own little world. Most of them seem to say in one way or another, "I'm the doctor, and I know what's best." They've been taught to think from a medical perspective, with little concern for the psychological. But they're finding out that the mind does have a lot of control over the body.

I don't hold doctors in reverence. I'm really handling the case. They can help, but it seems very important not to underestimate the body's ability to correct itself. The doctors are there for the times when it gets ahead of me. Like when I get pneumonia, I know that it will just get worse unless I have an aggressive antibiotic to kill it.

None of the doctors have ever put much emphasis on exercise, which is kind of strange, because I believe it's the major reason why I'm still here. It's the heart of my program. Girls do worse with CF than boys. I don't think scientists need to look for some technical explanation: It's probably because boys tend to be more active.

I've had my lungs collapse maybe five or six times, starting when

I was fifteen. After the first time, I would call the doctor or the hospital and say, "I have a collapsed lung." The doctors would say, "Oh, really," very skeptical that a patient would know what was going on with his own body. They would do an X-ray and, sure enough, it had collapsed. The doctors I have now seem to understand that I know more about my body than they do. After all, I've been living with it for more than thirty years.

I like my doctors; they ask for my input. When I was bleeding—I was hemorrhaging a lot—I called the doctor and suggested Vitamin K. He said, "Let's get a test done, but we'll start you on that even before the tests come back." He understood that I might know what was causing it. They respect my knowledge. I feel the doctors I have now really care.

Eight hours a day I'm in the best environment a person with CF could have. I'm a computer operator, and the computer room is climate controlled, 60 percent humidity, air-conditioned, no smoking. It's perfect. The concern isn't for the health of the employees, but fortunately the machines are very touchy and need to be in a stable atmosphere.

We have fun at work. We're in the operations room, and we're separated from the rest of the building. We have the music blaring, we're dancing around, so it's a lot of fun. I'm constantly moving, so I think it's the best job I could have.

In school, I was always the one making jokes, always laughing. At work now, I'm constantly laughing. I can be on the floor laughing. Laughing a lot is a big part of staying healthy.

People at work kid me. For lunch, I bring in potatoes and all kinds of vegetables—broccoli, carrots, asparagus, and meat, veal, and chicken and fish. Since I don't digest food well, the food I do get in has to be high in nutrients. So I don't eat any junk food. No potato chips or Whoppers.

I love eating. I think I have to. I'll get tired of it occasionally, but then I'll go out and have something special like some lobsters.

I eat four to five thousand calories every day. I don't gain weight. The big problem is not to lose any. If I get sick, I can drop down to 101, 102 in a couple of days. I don't want to get down that far because I haven't got that much to spare.

* * *

I'm not a social butterfly. I hate going out to dances or to bars. Because of my size and so forth, I feel that people are looking at me. I can't put up with the smoke. I used to tolerate it; now I won't. I'll ask them to stop, or I decide not go there anymore.

None of my friends smoke. It cuts out a lot of people who you may want to be friendly with, but if they're smoking, I'd rather not even talk with them.

Before people start to smoke, I wish they could spend a day inside my body, with my lungs, to see how I feel every day. It burns me up to see people who smoke. They're coughing; they have emphysema or cancer of the lungs. I can't quite believe it. Here they are with a normal body and they're doing this to themselves! And I have a problem that I didn't cause. I didn't ask for CF. I just don't get it!

I have a hard time understanding people who can't quit smoking, can't lose weight, can't stop drinking. Because every day, I have a routine that I can't waver from; I have to do therapy twice a day. I have to go out and run every night. I don't like doing it; I hate it. But if I want to live, I have to do it. It's constant maintenance.

My work has never been a problem for me. Relationships are a different story—sometimes I think it's simpler not to try.

I see someone cute and think, "Gee, I really should go up and say something." But then I ask myself, "Is it fair to get involved with someone if I'm not going to be around down the road?" I'm constantly battling with myself.

I question, can I afford the energy? A relationship takes a lot of energy.

I look back now on my first love. I was hanging on; I wouldn't let go even though the relationship was going bad. I didn't know what to do. I had backed out a number of times, but finally she made the decision, broke things up. That was that.

She couldn't talk about the CF. She crawled under a rock. I tried, but she just pulled back, dove for the nearest cover. How can you talk to someone who won't talk to you?

I was in love, and it made me crazy. I hurt a lot of people in my family over that relationship. I would go out, I'd drink, I'd come in late. Physically, it was damaging me. I got sick a lot. I put my parents through hell for a few years. They couldn't take it anymore. They almost threw me out of the house.

During this time, my parents went away to Bermuda for two weeks. I had a good time. I was drinking; I was staying up late. There was a lot of slippage with my routine. When they came back, they said that I looked like shit. I had deep dark circles under my eyes; I'd lost a lot of weight. I've learned that it's not worth the "good time."

I'm healthier when I'm not in a relationship. When I'm involved, I tend to neglect myself. I give more time to the person than is good for me. It becomes draining. I get sick. Maybe that's not a good relationship. A relationship is supposed to make you healthier, isn't it?

I think what keeps me going is the hope that there's someone or something out there that will be right for me. It's not about having a lot of money, because I have enough. Or a job, because that's all right. I think, it's the hope of getting to a place where I'll be happy.

OBSERVATIONS

Kurt's power, his physical and emotional power, originates from his ability to stay focused on his life task. Survival is the task, and near-perfect discipline is the vehicle. He subordinates everything else to this goal, realizing strength, meaning, and, at times, contentment in the process. There are no holidays for Kurt. With relentless determination, he struggles to understand what will be life giving, then vigilantly orients his behavior around these criteria. His food, his recreation, his sleep schedule, and ultimately even his choice of friends and lovers must be scrutinized according to how well they sustain his body. Survival dominates all other needs.

For Kurt, there can be nothing passive about living. The very act of breathing requires effort. Each day he must decide anew whether life is worth the struggle. If he simply becomes passive or complacent about life, he will soon die.

Paradoxically, accepting things as they are enhances the likelihood they will change. Behaviorist B. F. Skinner put it this way: "Nature to be commanded must be obeyed." Kurt lives by this principle, without any illusions about the limit of his command.

In order to comply with nature, with the demands of his body, he seeks to gain intellectual and visceral understanding. Equipped with an intimate familiarity with his heart and lungs, he works them as much as possible, but ultimately submits to their absolute authority. For example, he changed his workout routine when "the lungs decided they didn't like that." His language—he consistently speaks of "the" heart or "the" lungs—suggests the respect and knowledge he has for these parts of his body. He appreciates their independent functioning without losing sight of their interconnectedness.

Kurt's medical "success" is a partnership effort. He understands what conventional medicine has to offer and relies on its resources whenever appropriate. If he needs antibiotics to fight an infection or hospitalization to cope with a collapsed lung, he doesn't hesitate to call on his doctors for help. His dependence, however, is limited. It does not mean he relinquishes control of his treatment. Nor does he believe medicine will work any magic without his involvement. When he took the treadmill test, for instance, he did not helplessly wait to receive his score. He worked with the data, integrating it into his own refined understanding of his body. Objective quantitative measures give Kurt access to information about his body that might be difficult to ascertain intuitively. He is determined to push himself to the limit. Scientific medicine serves to inform him what these limits are.

The constancy of Kurt's physical efforts are remarkable. Day in and day out, he drives his body to the point of exertion that will yield the most beneficial results. He drives himself to the emotional edge as well. Through sheer force of will, he consciously shapes his feelings. He claims control over his emotional stance toward life: The decision to laugh or cry is his. And if he can't change his frame of mind directly, he might initiate an activity (for example, exercise that "kills the depression") to achieve a positive emotional state.

Kurt cannot afford to deny any aspect of his situation, for denial will distort the feedback he gives himself about his body—feedback he uses to make critical treatment decisions. Courageously he recognizes the unadorned physical reality. "The lungs are a bit worse off"; "the disease doesn't stop"; "a cold or flu could snowball." He is equally courageous when he acknowledges his deepest pain and greatest fears: He really wants to go out in the evenings after work; he wishes that he could plan a future; and the prospect of death is a frightening reality.

Admitting his fear serves him well. This kind of self-honesty is the best and perhaps the only meaningful preparation for life's uncertainties. When something difficult happens, as it eventually does to even the healthiest, fear will wreak havoc unless the individual has dared to embrace the fear. Michael Spinks, the only boxer ever to hold the title of Light Heavyweight Champion and then win the heavyweight championship, knows how devastating fear can be to one's body and mind. Before his 1988 fight with Mike Tyson, one of the century's most ferocious fighters, Spinks spoke with his seven-year-old daughter, Michelle. He told her:

> I'm scared of fightin' him, too; I look at that man and get bad dreams, same as you do. Only difference from anybody else who fights him is that I admit it. Go ahead, boy, I tell myself, smell and taste and feel it, lie down and roll in it. Shouldn't pretend you're not afraid if you are, Michelle; start off with one big lie like that on the ground floor and you're only gonna have to prop it up with more and more little ones to keep it standin'. One good punch, one bad wind, one hard knock in life, and that house of lies come tumblin' down, and all the fear you pretended not to feel beforehand gonna gang up and run through you like a pack of wild dogs.

Humor can be a powerful antidote for fear. Kurt, like many others who successfully cope with serious illness, uses humor to minimize the angst of existence. By making light of death through a shared joke, we know that we are not alone in our efforts to make sense of the absurdity of life. People who come to a cancer or AIDS support group for the first time are often surprised by the laughter. The following joke was warmly welcomed at one group I attended:

> A man who was very sick got the bad news from his doctor. The test had come back positive, and he was told that he would not even live to see another sunrise.
> He went home and told his wife the bad news. He said, "For old times' sake, let's make love one last time."
> His wife said she was sorry, but she was just too tired.
> The sick man persisted, "Come on. This is very important. I really want to."

The woman was not swayed, insisting that she was too exhausted.

Trying to persuade her, he went on, "Really, it'll be wonderful."

Unconvinced, she replied, "That's easy enough for you to say. You don't have to get up in the morning."

Kurt delights in life, but he is in a unique position to recognize its tragicomic nature. George Bernard Shaw summed it up well when he wrote, "Life does not cease to be funny when people die any more than it ceases to be serious when people laugh."

Intuition suggests that laughter is good medicine, but there is also scientific evidence that laughter produces specific physiological benefits.

During a good laugh, breathing becomes deeper and more spasmodic, heart beat and blood pressure increase. Marvin Herring, M.D., states "The diaphragm, thorax, abdomen, heart, lungs, and even the liver are given a massage during a hearty laugh." After the laugh, tension is released and blood pressure and heart rate, which had been elevated, fall below normal for about 45 minutes.

Laughing 100 to 200 times a day is equal to about ten minutes of rowing, according to William Fry, M.D., a psychiatrist at the Sanford Medical School. Laughter has also been associated with the body's production of endorphins. Endorphins are sometimes referred to as nature's opiates because of the feeling of euphoria associated with their release.

Kurt's desire to stay alive is so pervasive, his awareness of his body's needs so ingrained, that his subconscious helps get the job done. I found a similar pattern with each of our interviews. Initially he would be fully present and absorbed in the process. After about an hour and a half, Kurt would become restless and fidgety, and his concentration would suffer. When I asked him about my observation, he laughed. He said that whenever he sat for a while, regardless of how invested he might be, something inside would tell him to get up and move.

Kurt's body may imprison him, but the constancy of his physical needs also contains the seeds of his liberation. Survival is the source of meaning in his life, and survival demands that he live totally focused and fully conscious. Lapses in discipline are unforgiving. The option to sleepwalk through life, an option exercised regularly by many of us, is available to Kurt at only the steepest cost. Consequently practically all of his actions are deliberate and purposeful. Obviously there is much pain in his life, but he also knows the freedom of living a conscious and meaningful life.

Contemplating the transplant operation that may end his life is not merely a descent into hell; for rather than shifting the responsibility of choice to someone else, he remains totally involved and vital as he takes command of the decision-making process. There is no greater act of potency than initiating the decision that will make all the difference. Richard Leider, author of *The Power of Purpose*, explains the impact of immersion in a risky situation:

> Not only are our senses heightened and our emotions aroused but everything is focused on the successful completion of the experience. We can put our whole self into it. It is an enhancement of our life through testing ourself at the edge of growth. This is a way to live a healthy and satisfying life, to savor the challenges that expand our potential.

Unlike others, however, Kurt's risks are not limited to singular events like skydiving or mountain climbing. His entire life is lived on the edge, and he realizes both the limits and vast rewards of such a tenuous existence.

We can only speculate about the exact origin of Kurt's internal strength. He says his parents laid the foundation. Indeed, they lovingly demanded that their son adhere to the routine that would become his second nature. Their remarkable consistency would serve as an example for him in coming years, for parenting a chronically sick child is a difficult and demanding job. The natural desire is to make life as easy as possible for the child. Oftentimes, parents must choose between the child's immediate comfort and the child's well-being in the longer term. The Metzlers' willingness to persevere with what they believed was right served to model true discipline. The meta-message of their communication was not wasted on Kurt. Through their demands on him, they let him know that they were absolutely unambivalent—they loved him and wanted him to survive as long as possible.

While Kurt was growing up, the Metzler home was a haven, but the outside world was not so kind. He was different from the other children, smaller, barrel-chested, and with mottled teeth. Not an easy road for a child, not an easy plight for anyone. Yet he passed through the early years with his self-esteem intact. For his parents communicated that he was valuable, that he was loved. As he matured, these values were internalized. Feeling like a worthy person, he had reason to stay alive.

Once he entered adolescence, Kurt's parents had less influence and his peers more. It was not just coincidental, however, that he found Rossberg, a young mentor, who could reinforce the values he grew up with. Thus, he was spared a major and potentially deadly conflict of values with peers who could have inadvertently swayed him from his therapy, exercise, and diet to pursue the more "normal" adolescent stirrings of sex, drugs, and rock and roll.

Eventually he was able to transcend Rossberg's teachings. Rossberg's death, like the death of all his peers with CF, was not a reason to despair. It was used as a sign that he needed to strengthen his resolve.

As a child, Kurt was told he had to go out and play. More than just the literal message was taken in. He grew up knowing that life was to be played. Today he plays hard at everything. He strains to participate fully in life. Ironically, this desire presents yet another challenge, for Kurt cannot just give free reign to this boundless enthusiasm. His inclination to go all out, whether in sports or relationships, is potentially devastating. For many people who are ill, the major challenge is to find or rekindle a zest for life. Much of Kurt's work is to keep it from overflowing.

RELATED RESEARCH

Kurt understands that he must stay fully involved in all phases of treatment if he hopes to maximize his chances of survival. Although the extent of his medical involvement is considered highly unusual, Western medicine is beginning to recognize the value of including the patient on the treatment team. This evolution in medical thinking presents an irony, since healers throughout time have known the curative powers of the fully involved patient. Jerome Frank studied primitive cultures and found that patients frequently participated in planning their healing rituals. Often they do something for others, such as preparing a shared ceremonial meal. In this way, patients become participants in the recovery process, and, as Frank says, the activity can serve to "counteract their morbid self-absorption."

Contemporary research indicates a number of reasons for patients to become fully engaged in the treatment process:

1. The involved patient is more likely to adhere to necessary medical treatment, especially treatment that is painful or difficult. Industrial research has shown that authoritarian leaders will indeed get their followers to do what they say, but compliance is short-term. Workers who feel that their participation is discouraged miss work more often and are more likely to sabotage the efforts of the workplace. Research has demonstrated that having a choice can even improve performance. For example, subjects who can decide for themselves the order in which they will take various tests actually perform better than if they have no choice at all. There are many places in the medical setting where this knowledge could be transferred without financial cost and without compromising medical procedures.

2. A feeling of control may help the patient cope with the trauma of illness. Psychologists Ronnie Janoff-Bulman and Camille Wortman from the University of Massachusetts found that people paralyzed in freak accidents actually did better emotionally if they felt some responsibility for the accident. Such an attitude helped them to feel that they had more control over future accidents.

3. Feeling out of control may foster illness; taking control may facilitate healing. In one study, two groups of rats were subjected to electric shocks. Only one of the groups could make the shock stop (by rotating a wheel); the other group had no control. A reasonable hypothesis would be that the rats with the responsibility were subjected to more stress and would therefore suffer more physiologically. The results suggest otherwise. The rats who could not influence the outcome developed ulcers double the size of the rats with control.

Drs. Lawrence Sklar and Hymie Anisman implanted cancer cells in three groups of mice. The first group was exposed to electric shocks, but by moving into another compartment of the cage, they could avoid the shocks. The second group was subjected to shocks that they could not control. The third group was not shocked. The mice with no control developed the fastest-growing tumors and died the most quickly even though they were shocked for the same length of time as the mice with control. It's provocative to note that the rate of cancer growth for the rats that had control over their shocks was not any higher than for the shock-free group.

4. The action that the patient initiates may ease symptoms, slow the progress of a disease, and in some cases, lead to cure.

LEO PERRAS

God cures and the doctor sends the bill.

Mark Twain

My first interview with Leo Perras, more than six years ago, made me uncomfortable. He wore a large wooden cross, and crucifixes, statues, and pictures of Jesus were displayed about his house. Perhaps more unsettling than the religiosity was the realization that Leo's story did not fit, did not even come close to fitting, any of the psychological or medical models I was developing to explain extraordinary healing.

The facts seemed straightforward. While a young man, Leo was struck by a truck. A series of back operations left him a paraplegic. He was bound to a wheelchair for twenty years, with deteriorating health, until he went to a Catholic charismatic prayer service. During the service, Father DiOrio, a nationally known faith healer, told Leo to get up and walk. Leo did and has been walking since.

Because I could not dismiss Leo's story as unfounded or irrelevant, even after six years, I needed to meet with him again. The first task, however, was to determine conclusively the veracity of his account.

In the days that immediately followed his "cure," various magazines and newspapers cited Leo's physician as saying that his recovery was "truly a miracle"; his ability to walk was labeled a neurological

173

impossibility. The published reports also confirmed that Leo had neither reflexes nor sensations in his legs.

To verify the accuracy of the statements with the primary source of medical information, I attempted to reach his physician. After three registered letters and numerous phone calls, contact was finally made.

The reason for the doctor's reluctance became apparent. He began the conversation by saying, "I've given up on the guy. He has divorced his wife, and he thinks he has a mission. He wears a cross about eight inches long."

Despite the physician's disappointment with Leo's behavior, he did substantiate the extraordinary nature of the recovery:

> After 21 years in a wheelchair, his legs were wasted. His muscles were wasted. The legs were in very rough shape as testified to by the fact that he had a very serious infection in his foot. He had bought a new pair of shoes, just to wear in the wheelchair and there was a nail sticking up from the sole, but he never knew about it until his wife noticed this tremendous abscess on the ball of his foot. It was only after the foot swelled badly that the nail was found. So he had no sensation.
>
> Another time, he had a large perirectal abscess which he did not become aware of until it was far advanced. I was able to drain it, put drains in, with no anesthesia and absolutely no pain.
>
> For various and sundry reasons he required analgesics, heavy doses of all sorts of medication for years and years and years. Another amazing thing about this man is that suddenly, with this healing, he stopped taking everything. There was no withdrawal. He took nothing for pain, nothing for sleep. He didn't even take an aspirin. That's miraculous in itself.

Leo, aged 67, lived on a busy street, in a working-class neighborhood. As he had been on our first visit years before, Leo was waiting for me at the side door. On the way to the living room, I was impressed by the finely crafted pieces of woodwork throughout the house. The subtle detail and extreme care of his latest work, a mahogany table with a carved relief of the Last Supper, indicated that Leo was an expert woodworker. I commented upon its beauty, and Leo told me that the table, like most of the work, was to be a gift. Leo said a neighbor had admired a similar table in his shop. Since the man's birthday was coming up, Leo (who lived on Social Security) was making the table for his neighbor.

Leo was a small, thin man with glasses that seemed far too large for his face. But his voice was full and deep, his speech commanding and at times flamboyant. His manner was rough and so blunt that I did not fully appreciate what a compassionate and decent human being Leo was until after I had spent many hours listening to our taped conversations.

During this second visit, the artifacts around the room and the religious focus of his life no longer seemed an important barrier between us. In fact, the symbols of his belief felt quite natural. Since Leo had experienced an extraordinary force—whether it was the power of God or the power of his faith—it only seemed logical that he would want to express his gratitude and nurture this faith in every way possible.

He told me about his life:

My daughter and son-in-law were looking for a house, and they couldn't find one that they liked. So I said, "Get me a set of blueprints and I'll build you one."

My father is sitting there shaking his head, and he says, "You know, it's unfortunate nobody told you you're paralyzed."

I says, "Think about it a minute. It's not as impossible as you think. First of all, I don't think with my legs. Right?" So I says, "God gave me the talent to be a carpenter. I've got two hands to work with. If I can get next to it, I can do the work. So what's the big deal?"

He says, "You're going to go through with this, aren't you?"

I says, "Yup."

"Well," he says, "in that case, I'll give 'em the land for the house." Which he did.

Three weeks later, the project got off the ground. I built myself, for lack of a better word, a highchair. When the work got out of reach, they put me into it, and then I could reach the ceiling and do the work. And when it got to the roof part, they carried me up the ladder, and I'd do the work on the roof. At the end of the day, they'd take me back down.

The only mistake I made, I started at the end of September, I should have started in April, because it was a cold winter. One

Sunday, we were up on the roof shingling, and it started to snow and the snow was turning red all over the place. I'm telling my son-in-law, "What the hang's wrong?" He says, "It's you." I had opened up the whole hip from dragging on the shingles, bleeding all over the place. Of course, I didn't feel it. Well, they took me down from the roof, and that was that for a few days.

I got the house done in seven months. An accomplishment. A sign that I wasn't a useless individual, that I could still use my talent.

People would say, you're gonna build a house—you're crazy. You can't do it. But I could do anything I wanted, but walk.

My problems started when I was eighteen years old—got hit by a truck and was out of work for a year. Of course, before World War II, they didn't do disc operations as we know 'em. The solution then was a sacroiliac fusion. They put me in a body cast for several months, built up my left shoe to balance things out, and I wore a steel brace. There was a lot of pain.

Believe it or not, I was drafted soon after that. I was in the army seven weeks before they caught up with me in Illinois and discharged me. The colonel out there told me, "I would like to find the doctor who passed you. I'd have him on a rock pile for a while. But we did take you in, now we'll have to take care of you." And they sent me home.

I got married in 1945.

I was working on construction as a carpenter, heavy work, and I shouldn't have been doing it, I suppose, but that's my trade. Things got really bad in 1950.

I went to the VA hospital in Framingham, where they did a disc operation that seemed to be very successful. Three weeks later, an orderly came in on a Sunday night. This is an old military hospital, July and no air conditioning whatsoever. I had a heavy brace on with about an inch of felt padding inside. Hotter than blazes. So he came in on a Sunday night and says, "Leo, how would you like a back rub?"

I said, "That would be great." So he went over, got his paraphernalia, came back, and opened up the brace, and when he did, I started arching over backward. In other words, my head and my heels were trying to come together, and the pain was unbearable.

He ran out, got the nurse. The nurse came in, looked at me, and ran back to the nurses' station and called the doctor.

Being a weekend, they had an officer of the day who covered several wards. This man was an internist; he didn't know anything about orthopedics. He came in and looked at me. I'm praying to die, I can't handle it. So he gave me a shot and waited. There was no effect, so he gave me another shot, and it didn't work. Finally he told the nurse something, and she came back with a shot glass full of medication. They held my head and poured it down until I passed out.

The next morning, I opened my eyes about six o'clock, and this nurse was standing there. She said, "You awake?" And I nodded. She gave me another shot, knocked me right out.

I woke up around lunchtime. Two orderlies came in, strapped me to a stretcher, and brought me to a great big room. There were about twenty-five doctors and technicians in there, with my whole history on the blackboard. They're arguing back and forth; the orthopedic and neurosurgeons are arguing. The orthopedic men wanted to fuse ten vertebrae in my back; the neurosurgeons wanted no part of it because they felt they would have to go back in. The bottom line was that they were afraid that because the spasms in the back were so bad and causing so many degrees of arching, it would damage the spinal column.

They were worried about that. I was concerned with the pain; I can't handle the pain. Well, they settled on a nonsurgical approach.

That night, they took me up to the operating room, and this neurosurgeon put an intravenous in my arm. He gave me a pint of Procaine solution in my vein, to try and kill all this, to try and relax these muscles.

After a few minutes, the doctor is getting further and further away. I'm trying to talk and my tongue feels as though it is the size of a cucumber. He's laughing: "Well, at least it's working, but unfortunately it's only going to work for twenty-four hours."

They kept this procedure up for ten days before these spasms started to let go. A few weeks later, they sent me home, but I couldn't go to work. A year later, they let me go to work. And I went back to my woodworking.

In two years, I was back in the hospital, and they did another disc operation with a fusion. My right leg was partially paralyzed. Thirty-one days later, the doctor came into my room and said, "You're going home today. But before you do, I want to speak with you." So about ten o'clock I went to his office, and he told me that he assisted at the operation and didn't agree with the way it was done. He said I was going to end up with a lot of problems, worse than what I had. He said, "I'll be very blunt: You're going to end up in a wheelchair." Well, I didn't put too much stock in it.

Two months later, I went to work. Of course, I had my own cabinet shop, and things were going along pretty good.

But soon the pain started coming in again. At the least provocation, I'd fall flat on my face. It kept getting worse. Finally I got to a point where I didn't want to go into the shop; I was afraid that I would fall into the machines. I got very depressed and didn't talk to my wife or anybody else for over a month.

So my wife called a doctor, who came over to see me. Reluctantly— he's very nice about it—he suggested I go see a psychiatrist.

I said, "If that's what you mean, why didn't you come out and say so. You don't have to tell me I'm nuts. I know I am. All right? I've got problems. I can't handle it."

The first two sessions, I didn't talk. The third one, the psychiatrist says to me, "I noticed you don't sit in one place very long. You got back problems or something?" I thought to myself, oh my God, finally, he's going to get to it. I started telling him about it.

He said, "Why didn't you tell me about this before?" He picked up the phone, called a neurosurgeon from Springfield: "I want you to see this man; he needs help, and he needs it now."

I think it was four days later, I went down, and the surgeon examined me and he says, "You're a mess." So he wrote to the VA for some records, and he didn't get anything back that he wanted. He contacted 'em again. Finally he says to me, "Who operated on you? Nothing is signed here."

I says, "I have no idea."

He says, "What are you talking about?"

I says, "It was a doctor from Boston. I don't know who he is. I never spoke to him in my life."

"That's a hell of a way to run things."

I says, "That's the way the VA is."

He decided he's going to do a myelogram. Monday morning, there's forty litters in the hallway, and everybody goes in and that's it. He did the myelogram, and he couldn't get anything through the lower part of the back. There was a blockage. He says to me that the only thing he could do was an exploratory to try and find out what the problem was.

A month later, they did the operation. I woke up, and I was paralyzed from the ribs down.

Needless to say, that was the end of the world. I'm laying there, my youngest daughter is a year and a half, the oldest one is twelve, I've got five kids. You lay there wondering, afraid, what's going to happen now?

The doctor wouldn't come near me. He thought we were going to blame him. My wife and I had discussed it. We knew there was the possibility this could happen. I wasn't blaming him for this. I just wanted some answers. What happened? Nobody was giving me the answers.

For five days, he wouldn't come near me until my wife called up and read him the riot act.

They all said I would never walk again, and they thought that the sooner I got used to it, the better.

The first two or three weeks in the hospital, thoughts crossed my mind, "What have I done to deserve this? How can I live like this?" You know, this self-pity business.

Thirty days later, I came home. I didn't want to go anywhere. I didn't want to be seen. For two months, I didn't leave the house.

After the initial shock, most people will really have to make a decision: Can you live with it? That is the question.

I lay there, and a million things ran through my mind. Sooner or later, I knew I had to come to a decision. I could either dwell in my self-pity or go out and do something with my life. Gradually I decided that this is the way I had to live.

I developed the attitude that I could be worse off. Everybody has problems, one way or another. Nobody has a monopoly on problems. Some are more visual than others, but like I used to tell other paraplegics, "The guy you envy walking down the street may have cancer. And he may not be around six months from now. So tell me about it."

There was no point in envying everybody else, because with that attitude, you only destroy yourself. I've seen this happen with many paraplegics. They can't handle it, and they end up committing suicide.

Twenty years ago, things were quite different for handicapped people than they are today. You had to fight your way—no ramp curbings, no parking spaces reserved for the handicapped. Everything was a great accomplishment. I no longer took things for granted. Before, I used to go over a curb twenty times a day and never give it a thought, but suddenly it could've been a ten-foot wall to me. I never said too much about it because I figured I was one of a very, very small percentage of the citizens of this town. Why should they have to turn the town upside down for me? I never wanted anyone to cross the street because they saw me coming. I never wanted to be a pain in the neck to anyone.

It used to bother my mother a great deal that I was paralyzed. I would tell her, "Thank God for the wheelchair so I can get around, hand controls in the car so I can drive. Suppose that I was in bed twenty-four hours a day, and that's possible." You've got to count your blessings. I can do a little woodwork. Never mind, I can't do this, I can't do that.

I was asked to get out of a restaurant because they said I was cluttering the place up with a wheelchair. The owner came over and said, "What are you coming in here for, cluttering this place up?" It hurt.

It happened to me twice. They wouldn't dare do it today. But I says that's just the way human beings are. They're not aware of other people's feelings. And once it has been said, all the apologies in the world . . . forget it! It's been said. You can't take it back.

People who I thought were good friends, once I got paralyzed, I never saw them again. This cut deep. People use the term "friend" very loosely. Now I realize, if you have one or two friends, good friends, in a lifetime, then you are a millionaire. This has happened all over again with this divorce. People who I thought were good buddies of mine I haven't seen in three or four years.

I'm adjusting. A year goes by, and I develop this pain again. I went to a neurosurgeon who said, "A good percentage of you paraplegics develop intractable pain from the nerve roots. Not a hang of a lot you can do about it." He suggested I go to Boston, which I did.

I went back to the VA, and they did all kinds of nerve blocks trying to stop the pain. They decided to do a cordotomy, where they go in your neck and cut away part of the spinal cord, hoping to stop the pain. I came out of that, but I couldn't use my left hand, my left eye was closed, I couldn't urinate because it affected the bladder and kidneys, and I'm shooting temperatures every afternoon, out of sight. And I said to the chief of the ward, "What's going to happen now?"

He says, "There's nothing more we can do for you." Well, thanks for nothing.

They sent me home, and I was in bed for ten months. I darn near gave up on that one. By then I was praying, if I could just get back in the wheelchair. You know, your attitude changes.

I had two choices—to go in a corner and cry, or to go out and live. Again I decided that this was the way I had to live.

I was having trouble with the wheelchair because my left hand was so bad. You can't get up a ramp with one good hand. Finally I started getting around a little bit.

You can get to feeling pretty useless. I had a family, and I should be supporting them. But who was going to hire me?

So I took this job as a volunteer at Cooley Dickinson Hospital. I was doing messenger work, printing and whatnot.

The woman who was in charge of my department kept watching me. I'd been there about six weeks when one afternoon she handed me a job application.

I said, "Don't waste my time. Nobody wants to hire a paraplegic." She says, "Fill it out, will ya!"

I said, "All right."

Three o'clock, I went to leave for my last rounds for the day. She says, "You're not going to do these rounds. The controller wants to talk with you." So I went in to talk with the controller.

I said, "I've never worked in an office before. I'm a cabinetmaker."

He says, "I know that. I've been checking you out. Cabinetmakers are notorious for details. You're the man I'm looking for. How about starting tomorrow?"

As I'm going out the door, I says, "What am I going to be doing anyway?"

He says, "I want you to supervise that whole section."

I looked at him. "You've got to be kidding."

He said, "You can handle it."

I told him. "I haven't been to high school."

He says, "I'm surrounded by educated idiots. I can't get anything done. That's the truth. I want somebody who can go out there and get it done. All right?"

"All right."

Well, the first month I was tempted to give it up forty times. I was used to working alone as a cabinetmaker or on construction. Now I was supervising sixteen women. They were driving me nuts. The men would tell you where to go when they didn't like something. Never mind this fancy business.

I finally got the hang of it. We organized the three departments I was in charge of, and things went along pretty good. My boss kept handing me more and more work. He used to say, "We use the path of least resistance. I know if I give it to you, it'll get done."

He started coming around with me. He said, "This is unbelievable. These people never look at you when you talk; they look at the ceiling."

I said, "I know, I'm observant enough to realize that." I never wanted to be pitied. I wanted to be accepted like anybody else. They felt uncomfortable, so you had to take the initiative and say, "Hey! There's a person between these wheels. I'm a human being. I think like everybody else. I have the same desires. I just use a different method of getting around." Pretty soon you get to realize which people are uncomfortable around you. Even some of the nurses were. You have to take the initiative to make 'em feel comfortable.

They kept throwing more and more work at me. But being handicapped I was expected to do more than others, to prove a point. The pressure was there. After a year, I came down with a bleeding ulcer that was serious.

My boss felt bad. He thought he had been giving me too much work, and he says, "I've been pushing too much at ya." He promised to lighten up the load.

In between my work, I'm talking to patients with problems to try and help them out. To me they couldn't say, "I'm stuck in a wheelchair, what the hell do you know."

I was on the East Wing one morning to check out a machine that wasn't working. The head nurse says to me, "Do you know Mr. Chapin?" I says, "Not personally." She says, "He's in the last private room on the right. I want you to go down and talk with him. Short of throwing him out bodily, you have my permission to do whatever you have to do. He's an ornery old cuss."

So I go down there and start talking to him. I says, "What the hell ya doing in bed."

He snarls his lip and snaps, "Can't walk."

I says, "I can't either." So I start, "So you're the guy I sent that brand-new wheelchair to last week. I understand you're a self-made man, you ended up chairman of the board of the bank. What did you do with that man, leave him at home? Put him in a closet somewhere? Don't you have the guts to get out of bed and get in that wheelchair and go out and live?"

He said to me, "You don't know who you're talking to!"

"Why," I said, "are you someone special?"

He says, "I happen to be chairman of the board of trustees of this hospital."

"Oh. Does that mean my job is in jeopardy?" I told him, "I've got news for you, I don't care if I work here tomorrow or not. How's that grab ya?"

He starts to say "You lousy son of a . . ." But I interrupt him. "Mr. Chapin, I've been in this wheelchair for years. Don't tell me what it's about. I know what it's about. Think about it." And I leave his room.

The next morning, I come down from Medical Records, he's out in the hall in his wheelchair. I says to him, "Does the nurse know you're here?"

He says to me, with his lip still snarled, "I'm not accustomed to asking; I'm accustomed to giving orders. I do what I want! You made a lot of statements yesterday. Today I want some answers. Come on in." So we talked.

The day after that, he comes out with a bright plaid sport coat and his racing cap. He's all dressed up, and I ask him where he was going. He says, "Well, we spent several hundred thousand dollars beautifying the grounds. I'm going out to smell the roses."

They called it ministry work in those days. It was just being concerned with others and their problems.

The following year, I spent seven weeks in the hospital again. Ulcers. I'm mulling the whole thing over, and I says to my doctor, "This is it."

"What do you mean?"

I says, "I'm going back to woodworking. I never had ulcers doing woodworking."

So I spoke with my boss, "I've had it with this job. First of all, they don't want to pay me what I should be getting." I says, "I find some of the people I'm supervising are getting more money than I am." I had done the budgets that year for the business office, so I knew what was going on. They didn't think they had to pay me more because I was in the wheelchair. And I says, "I don't appreciate it." My boss wanted to get me the money, but the higher-ups wouldn't go along with it.

After I built my daughter's house, I went into my shop and broke up the cement floor. I built forms and repoured concrete and left some pits so I could drop my machines. Because they were up too high, they were under my chin. I built an addition and put an elevator in the shop so I could get up and down stairs. I came up with all kinds of inventions, hydraulic lifts and whatnot, so I could work and do what I wanted.

I decided that since this is the way I've got to live, let's make it as easy as possible. It was a challenge. I accepted the challenge. My kids always said the word "impossible" was not in my vocabulary. And it wasn't. Nothing's impossible, if you sit down and think about it. There's always a way of doing things.

When things settled down a bit, I organized a company, Tasks Unlimited. We had ten people working there for a while. The only criterion: You had to be handicapped. It was an uphill battle all the way. You'd go into these plants and before you could even open your mouth, they'd tell you, "We don't need anything today," assuming you were looking for donations. But this was strictly competitive.

I had four partners. They assumed that you'd get work because you were in a wheelchair. That was not a fact. So I decided to pull out and let them take over.

During this time, because of the cordotomy, the whole left side of the chest and my left arm was deteriorating. The muscles were dying out because they had severed the nerves.

Spring of '78, I started in with pain that was so bad I couldn't handle it. I had bilateral Ménière's, inner ear problems. I was back on Demerol and Percodan and whatnot for pain. Then I came down with arthritis; I couldn't get out of bed in the morning. I came down with gallbladder problems.

My doctor said to me, "Leo, I don't know what to do with you anymore. Medically we've about reached the bottom of the barrel. Every week, something gets worse." And I told my youngest daughter, "I'm not going to see Christmas this year. Not the way things are going. No way."

Well, Dr. DiOrio—I mean Father DiOrio had come into Holyoke, ten minutes from home, in April, and I refused to go. I wanted no part of it. I knew nothing about him, never heard of him before.

My doctor was trying to get me to go. He had sent his wife to get some tickets. My wife said, "You know, you're going to hurt their feelings by doing this."

I said, "I don't care. If God wants to heal me, he can heal me right here."

I had so much pain, I didn't want to go anywhere. I'm on 2 ccs of Demerol, and I'm taking eight or nine Percodans a day, and I'm on sleeping medication. Two or three nights in a row, there'd be no sleep. I just could not relax because the pain would never stop.

All summer long, my wife and friends would casually mention Father DiOrio. I heard stories, but I don't believe everything I hear because some people exaggerate, it's human nature. I don't fault anyone for that, but as a cabinetmaker I always dealt in concrete things. You could see it cr you couldn't.

There was no big pressure to go. My wife knew me. It wouldn't do any good because I can be very stubborn. I wasn't involved in the conversations. "Don't bother me with it," was my attitude.

On Saturday night, she got hold of my best buddy. August 26, he called me up and says, "Father DiOrio's having services in Worcester tomorrow. We're going."

I says, "Good. I hope you enjoy it."

He says, "We're going, and you're coming with us."

I said, "I'm not going anywhere." We didn't really argue, but more or less talked about it over the phone. He wasn't giving an inch. He was very insistent. Then I says, "All right, if that'll make you happy, I'll go."

You know, I wasn't a martyr. If there was an out, I'd have taken it. Some people enjoy their problems, but I didn't. I just didn't think it would do any good.

I got up the next morning, and I was grumpier than blazes. I cleaned out the van and threw some pillows in the back because I figured I'd be tired when I got home. I'd sleep on the way back.

We left about 11:00, picked up some friends of ours. Seven of us went down. My wife was praying for me to get rid of pain. I went down with the specific intention of praying for my youngest daughter. She was having marital problems, and that bothered me. My plan was to find a comfortable little corner in the church where I wouldn't bother anybody.

I couldn't believe it when I got there. The street was jammed with people. There were ten, twelve policemen trying to control the crowd. I says to my buddy, "This is unusual. Did you ever see people fight to get in church before?"

He said, "No. It must be something different here." I couldn't believe it.

Finally they separated the crowds so I could get through. They brought me up eight or nine steps into the church, and the ushers immediately told us that all wheelchairs go up in front. My wife is sitting in the first pew right next to me. I looked at her and says, "My God, you can't get lost in this place. They stick you right up front." I wanted to dissolve in the crowd and forget about it.

The church was jammed to the doors. Three o'clock, this Father DiOrio came out, started the service. He always started by anointing members of the ministry. These are people that sing in the choir or that usher. As he's anointing these people with oil, they're falling all over the floor! I'm looking at this and saying to myself, "What the hell did you get into here?" I'm watching the service with reservations. I was brought up a Catholic, but this was different.

About six o'clock, I looked at my wife, and she knew that I was getting ready to leave. The pain was so bad I couldn't handle it.

All of a sudden he comes out in front of the altar: "We've had many healings here this afternoon. We pray and thank God for that.

What we need now is something more visual. I want everybody to get with prayer." He said, "Now don't fool around!"

What I didn't know was that on Thursday, the man who records the service said to Father DiOrio, "Father, what's your problem. I notice you never go near wheelchairs. You don't do the healing. God does the healing. What are you afraid of?"

I also found out later that I was the first one he looked at that day, and he couldn't get me out of his mind.*

You could hear a pin drop in that place. He picks his head up, and he says, "Something magnificent is about to happen like we have never seen."

I push myself up on my elbows, and I look at my wife and says, "This one I've got to see."

When he gets through talking, he turns around, takes the holy water off the altar and walks right up to me. He blesses me with the holy water, says a prayer, and puts his hand out. "In the name of Jesus Christ, rise," and before I realize what's happening, I'm standing for the first time in twenty years. I am literally picked up out of the chair.

I only knew that I was standing when it hit me that I was face to face with him. I had tried this forty million times in the last twenty years.

He says to me, "I want you to bend down and touch your toes." My first thought is: You're going to fall flat on your face. I had no muscles left; my legs were all atrophied. Without hesitation, I go down, touch my toes, and straighten back up, no problems whatsoever. The pain is gone, totally gone. Split second.

He says, "How long have you been in that wheelchair?"

"Twenty years, two months."

"You and I are going to walk down the center aisle of this church to the front doors and back." He starts walking backward and I follow him. My wife is petrified. She can't even move! The guy behind her says, "He's still walking."

She says that she can't move. So he picks her up by the shoulders and turns her around.

---

*In *The Man Beneath the Gift*, Father DiOrio says, "I had never seen him before that day. But as soon as my eyes fell on him, I felt as if a magnet was drawing me to him. Next thing I knew I was standing beside his wheelchair, looking down at him."

I walk all the way to the front of the church, turn around, and come all the way back.

My buddy is sitting about halfway down the aisle. He gets up on a pew to see if it's me. When he realizes who it is, he starts shouting at the top of his lungs, and crying, and everything else. His wife keeps trying to tell him we're in a church. You cannot shut the guy up, he's so happy.

I get back and kneel down at the sanctuary. I bet I'm there twenty minutes trying to get my composure back. My wife is asking herself, is he going to be able to get up? Pretty soon I kneel up straight, get up, and walk back. She says, "How do you feel?"

I say, "The pain is gone. Everything is gone."

She says, "You must be tired. Why don't you sit down?"

"I've been sitting for twenty years. No way I'm going to sit down." I stood up for the rest of the service. I felt as though I could fly. I came out of there pushing my own wheelchair. It's great to be walking, but to me the greater thing was to be without pain for the first time in thirty years or so. It's never come back.

When we got back to town that night, I went right to my doctor's house. There were seventeen or eighteen of us by then. We pulled up in front of the house, and my wife rings the doorbell. The light went on, and the good doctor opens the door. He was barefooted, had a robe on; he was getting ready for bed. He looked at me and grabbed his head. He says, "Oh my God!"

We went inside, and he started checking me over. After he's finished, he says, "You know, medically you don't have anything to walk with. You don't have any reflexes; you don't have any muscles; you don't have anything. I saw you walk in here, but that's medically impossible. But I have to believe what I see."

He said, "To try and make you people understand how great this is, you take a normal person who has fallen and broken a leg. You take 'em to the hospital, set the leg, and depending upon the injury, it's five, six, or seven weeks in a cast. You remove the cast, then you send 'em to physiotherapy, give 'em a pair of crutches and teach 'em how to walk again." He says, "This man hasn't walked for twenty years, all kinds of neurological problems, yet he gets up and walks immediately. That's medically impossible."

When I walked into my house, the phone was ringing. It was the doctor. He said, "I can't sleep, and you're not going to sleep either." So ten minutes later he and his wife came over.

One person was calling another, "Did you hear what happened to Leo Perras?" The first thing they'd ask, "What did he die from?"

The next morning, I woke up and laid there asking myself, Is this reality? Is this a dream or did it really happen?

I got up, no problems.

Then the newspapermen started coming in, and the photographers. The house was filled with people by eight A.M. For days, there was no time to eat or think.

I asked myself, "Why me? A nincompoop like me, who am I? You know, a woodworker; I never set the world on fire." People say to me, "I'm not worthy of being healed." Well, I'm not either when you get right down to it.

Of course, it was difficult to accept that I'm walking because I couldn't feel the floor under me; I didn't have any feeling. It was like being suspended in air. I kept looking down, and the feet were working but there seemed to be no connection between the mind and the floor. When I'd go up stairs, I'd have to check to see if my feet were on the right step. Yet everything was working. It was very hard to adjust to this. The pain never came back. The arthritis was gone. I never had any more trouble with my gallbladder.

The druggist said I would go into withdrawal for six months because of the medication I was on. For nine years, I had been taking eight or nine Percodans a day, which is addictive. Demerol is addictive; I was on Seconal trying to get some sleep. The druggist says, "I don't know about the rest of this, but this no withdrawal business blows my mind." The ear specialist I saw said, "You shouldn't be able to walk because you don't have any equilibrium." I said, "Well, I do a pretty good imitation of it." The neurosurgeon had something else to be amazed about.

People used to ask me, "Doesn't it bother you? Maybe tomorrow morning you can't walk?" My question to them: It doesn't bother you? You don't have a guarantee of the next minute.

One of my aunts called me up, very emotional. She told me it was too bad it was only going to last seven days. I asked her, "Where is this coming from?" She told me it was the general consensus in the building where she lives. I said, "Are you telling God what he's going to do?" A buddy of mine was more generous;

he gave me thirty days. I says, "Don't hold your breath. All right!" They're not counting anymore. It's been nine years in August.

As time went along, I got progressively better. Then, when the feelings started coming back, it began to make some sense. It was great when I could feel the pavement under my feet. Within a space of three months, all the feeling came back, the muscles came back, and things kept getting gradually better. But it was very mind boggling to try and take it in and analyze it. You know, some clergymen say to me, well, it was a case of self-hypnosis. I says, "You call it whatever you want." I've had other people tell me it was a momentary surge of adrenaline.

I lived for twenty years in that wheelchair. I was the one who had all that pain. Nobody else. I says, "You have a right to your opinion, but don't tell me what it's all about. I know where I've been, and I know where I am today. There's only one that gets credit for it: That's the Lord—period." Everything the medical profession tried to do made it worse. Three operations, believe me, it wasn't worth it. I says, "Thanks a lot for nothing." One doctor says to me, "I'm amazed you're still talking to us." Well, what can you do?

People ask me, "Do you suppose those nerves they severed are connected?" I says, "Personally I don't care, because I feel good." But I was working out back one day. My wife came over, looked at me, and started to laugh. She said, "Nothing has really changed."

I said, "What are you talking about?"

She said, "Look at yourself." I looked down. Only half of me was wet with perspiration, the other half perfectly dry. After they did the cordotomy, I never perspired from the left side of my body. So the condition still exists. So how do you explain it? I don't try.

Some are healed, and some are not. Father DiOrio says, "I don't do the healing. I don't have the answers." I've known people who have gone to Worcester eighty times since this happened—nothing has happened to them. I think in some cases it may be faith. But not in other cases. I went reluctantly. God will choose certain persons in spite of themselves. How do you explain a young child who suddenly gets healed. Faith has nothing to do with it.

A certain number of these things are going to be psychosomatic. But let's say a person is a hypochondriac, and then suddenly they no longer have their complaints. Well, that's also a healing.

Of course, my buddy from Springfield kids around with me. He said I was healed because I have a big mouth, and I would spread it all over the world.

Unfortunately—well, unfortunately or not unfortunately—people chose to put me on a pedestal, that I was no longer a human being, that I didn't have feelings like other people, I didn't think like other people: "Oh my God, don't tell me you're here. You're going to come into my house?"

"Hey, wait a minute. This is ridiculous. I still do woodwork. I still do the things I did before." People sometimes have an attitude about me that has nothing to do with me. I never felt better than anyone else. And when I was in the wheelchair, I never felt worse than anyone else.

When I got divorced, some people couldn't handle it. They said I was Catholic, I shouldn't've done it.

A year after the healing, I was really taken up in ministry work. The limelight was on me, not because I wanted it, but because of the circumstances. I was trying to get my wife involved, too, but she didn't want it. After living a quiet life of a woodworker and being in a wheelchair for twenty years, I was not that comfortable being projected into the limelight. But I also thought that people needed to know that these kinds of things are still happening. Like Father DiOrio says, "Shout it from the rooftops!" To do this, you are involved with TV programs and traveling. I've been out to Kentucky twice for a week at a time, been down to Florida, been all over. This started problems.

My wife accused me of running around, and it was not a fact. I says, "How could you misinterpret the work I'm doing to think that I'm running around with women?"

I talked to a priest about it. "The problem," he says, "is that she is used to being in the driver's seat for twenty years while you were in a wheelchair. She likes the driver's seat. She doesn't want to take the backseat. It's going to cause problems." And it did. It went from bad to worse and ended up in divorce, which is unfortunate. But it wasn't tolerable anymore.

But I didn't take it lightly. Like this priest says to me, he says, "There is a fine line between love and hate." And he says, "When it gets to hate, then we are talking about your salvation, my friend. So, when you can't resolve it, get out. Let's be realistic about the whole situation," he says. "After listening to your wife, it's going to get worse. My suggestion to you is to do something about it," which eventually I did. But it wasn't a good situation.

The limelight has brought other complications. I was having breakfast in a restaurant a few months ago. A young fellow sat down next to me. He kept looking over until he says, "I know you. I saw you on television."

I says, "Good. That and fifty cents will get you a cup of coffee."

He says, "You know, the devil works through DiOrio, too."

I thought, Oh cripes, I've got a Jehovah on my hands. I said, "I'm afraid you're being misled, young fella."

"Why?"

I said, "The Apostles didn't perform miracles. God performed the miracles, all right."

He said, "Your theory is all wet."

I said, "Well, you brought it up, so I'll give you my point of view. I don't know where you get your information, but you're wrong. The devil will never heal in the name of Jesus Christ. I got news for you, that does not happen. He will not give glory to God."

And he said, "Well, maybe."

"You may say maybe, I have no doubts. I know where it's coming from." I said, "Your theory doesn't hold any water. I didn't bring it up, you did." So that was the end of the conversation. I had to get my licks in.

You see, Father DiOrio is just the instrument being used to show the power of God. He can use any of us. Father DiOrio couldn't cure the wart on a frog. And he feels the same way.

I was invited to meet with some people. I thought they wanted this priest to talk with me, when all this time they really wanted me to talk to him. Anyway, this priest was dodging the question all evening. He's going on and on about Shakespeare and this and that. Finally this guy's wife stopped him and she says, "Father, I'm going to put it to you point-blank. What is your opinion about what happened to Leo?"

He says, "I'll be very honest with you. DiOrio is running a circus in Worcester; he ought to knock it off. And all the people who go there are a bunch of kooks."

I looked at him and said, "Are you calling me a kook?"

"Yea."

"That doesn't surprise me a bit, coming from you," I said. "We've been sitting here talking for over two hours, and you have been quoting Shakespeare and Milton by the mile. Did you ever hear of the Bible? What is your ministry here as a priest? Will you explain that to me? You don't believe that God can heal people today? If you don't, you got problems. You missed the boat altogether."

I finished by saying, "I'll tell you what I'll do, when I go home tonight, I'll pray for you."

When you get right down to it, you can't criticize someone for lack of faith. Because faith is a gift from God. Some have it, some don't. Like I said to him, I'll pray for you. That's about all you can do.

OBSERVATIONS

After leaving Leo's, I picked up my six-year-old son from kindergarten and headed home. I asked him about his day; he asked me about mine. Driving along, I briefly told him Leo's story, I finished by saying that I didn't really understand what had happened. My son, however, wasn't perplexed. Before racing off to play with his friends, he let me know, "Dad, it was a miracle."

Indeed, maybe it was as simple as that. Perhaps God had intervened through Father DiOrio to cure Leo's paralysis, take away his pain, and eliminate any physiological or psychological dependence on narcotics. Depending upon one's worldview, healing is a terribly complex or a very simple phenomenon. The explanation that follows is not more valid than Leo's. It's just a different way of making sense of the world.

The premise is that tremendous power can be derived from one's beliefs. Somehow faith enables the individual to mobilize the most extraordinary inner resources, making phenomenal physical cures possible. The power of faith—the belief that recovery is possible and probable—has been known since the dawn of medicine. Indeed, we don't know how Leo was cured, but many events converged that could have potentiated the full power of his belief system.

Leo tells us that he went to the charismatic renewal service with meager expectations and little knowledge of Father DiOrio. He was skeptical, but he wasn't totally closed. Even though travel was difficult, he thought there was enough potential to make a trip. He also went with the intention of praying for his daughter's marital peace—not as spec-tacular as a physical cure, but a difficult enough request to show that he had at least a shred of hope. His belief may have approached the way some people feel just before they blow out their birthday candles. They don't really think the wish will be granted, but, just in case, they make the wish rather than "blowing off" the possibility of a long shot coming through. Leo went to the service with a kernel of faith, and, as Jesus said, faith the size of a mustard seed, the smallest of all seeds, is all that one needs.

The people who were closest to him in the world nurtured whatever faith Leo did have. Their words and actions communicated that some-thing positive could come from the trip to see Father DiOrio. His doctor got him the tickets and his best friend insisted he attend, all the while his wife plugged the latent benefits of the service.

Months before Leo attended the service in Worcester, Father DiOrio had conducted one just minutes away from Leo's home. Not making this easy trip may have been fortuitous, for we often attribute the greatest power to the most foreign. Leo's eventual trip wasn't that far, but it replaced his everyday surroundings with a novel setting, creating a new opening. The unknown holds the promise that anything is possible; expectations of the greatest magnitude are stimulated. Bernie Siegel says that he seems to have the most medical success with people who have traveled the farthest to see him. It's interesting to note that, according to the New Testament, Jesus could not cure anyone in his own town.

Also consider Lourdes, France, celebrated for its miraculous cures. Since 1858, the Roman Catholic Church has officially cited sixty cases as miraculous; since 1954, thirteen miracles have originated there. After investigating these cases, the International Medical Committee of Lourdes calls them "scientifically inexplicable." Each year more than 500,000 people make the pilgrimage; despite the ordeal of the journey, the experience often improves their condition. Yet no one who lives near Lourdes has ever experienced a miraculous cure. Bathing in the spring, praying at the shrine, as well as the hardship of the trip to Lourdes are all necessary components of the "treatment."

When Leo arrived at the church, many events nurtured the suspension of his belief system. Nothing was as usual. After spending twenty years in a wheelchair, Leo was accustomed to second-class treatment. Maintaining respect from others was a constant struggle. At the church, however, he was suddenly treated like a guest of honor; a path was cleared for him, and he was ushered to the front.

The scene at the church—people fighting to get in—was entirely alien to his experience. Leo states that he couldn't believe it, while his friend confirms that this church is indeed something different from anything they have previously known. Jerome Frank, who has studied miracles and primitive healing, attributes the remarkable results, again at such places as Lourdes, to the expectation of cure. Miracles become credible as they are discussed and thought about constantly: Hope is everywhere.

To effect a cure, Father DiOrio uses all the resources at his disposal, including the power of suggestion. He frequently begins the service by saying, "As I walk among you, some of you will feel electricity going through you right out of my body. Heat. A jolt of lightning, so to speak. I don't know how God does it. Curvatures of the spine will begin straightening out. Bent legs will begin to straighten. We will probably see shortened legs begin to grow. These are the ailments which seem to be healed in every service. Other ailments—cancer, blindness, or paralysis, for example—seem to be healed in clusters."

During the service, Father DiOrio explains what "falling under the power" means. His description not only provides information, it increases the likelihood that congregation members will in fact "fall under the power." He tells the congregation, "Some of you will be falling down, or entering a state of divine spiritual ecstasy. What happens when someone falls or enters a standing ecstasy is an . . . overpowering of the spirit. The Lord usually likes to pass through people. . . . The saints used to experience this type of prayer; it's called 'ecstatic union.' They were just lost in God. Their bodies, with their external senses, became suspended, and they would just float in the Lord. You have no control. . . ."

His communication is stylistically similar to the way a therapist induces a hypnotic trance in a patient. The language is different, but Father DiOrio, like a hypnotherapist, encourages individuals to let go of their conscious or sensory awareness. He suggests the person's body may feel very light, and the usual relationship with the senses may be released. Again, like a skilled therapist, there is nothing coercive about his approach; he gives the individual a choice about whether or not to give up control. He lets congregation members know, though, that there is little reason to resist giving up their power, for it is highly pleasurable, an "ecstatic union" with God. Father DiOrio encourages them to let go of conscious awareness so they can tap into a wondrous source of power. For the priest, the source of power is God, while the therapist often speaks of one's inner power—the vast potential of the unconscious.

Father DiOrio had been primed for someone in a wheelchair. He confirmed that on the day of the service a member of his ministry told him not to be afraid of the people in the wheelchairs, reminding him that God, not Father DiOrio, did the healing. The climax was set when Father DiOrio told everyone to get with prayer and then Leo, a paralyzed woodworker, was chosen from among the hundreds of people who filled the church well beyond its capacity. Father DiOrio approached Leo and commanded him to get up and walk.

Certainly in the years of Leo's paralysis no one ever commanded him to walk. No one believed it was possible. For the first time in twenty years, someone—not just anyone, but the person who was the conduit for ultimate authority and knowledge—communicated absolute confidence that he could, that he would walk.

After his walk down the church aisle, a series of events minimized the likelihood that he would return to a life of paralysis and pain. As soon as he got up from his wheelchair, his life was irreversibly changed: He now knew that something he had tried a million times before was indeed possible. At some level, familiar contexts perpetuate continuity of roles. Suddenly the context in which he had lived—a paralyzed person with deteriorating health—disappeared. He became the subject of intense curiosity and, for some, reverence. The media attention and his new involvement with the church, as well as the obvious physical benefits, were all positively reinforcing.

Even if factors did converge to release the full power of Leo's faith, a question arises: Can faith really invest the body with extraordinary power?

Leonard Feinberg, Ph.D., chronicled a Sri Lanka firewalking ceremony in the May 1959 issue of the *Atlantic Monthly*. Since he had been a Fulbright Professor at the University of Ceylon [Sri Lanka] in 1956 and 1957, he had ample opportunity to explore the ritual. The firewalk culminated three months of rigorous religious preparation. The object of the walker's prayer, meditation, fasting, and religious instruction was direct communion with Kataragama, the local god. If the walker achieved complete faith in him, the fire could do no harm.

On the evening of the ceremony, hardwood logs filled a pit more than twenty feet long and six feet wide. Once the wood burned to a deep bed of charcoal, the pit was ready. But the exact moment would come only when the walkers felt united with Kataragama. Priests and students flowed directly from the nearby temple to the pit. Because of the intense heat, Feinberg said it was difficult for him to stand closer than ten feet from the coals. Recorded temperatures inside the pits typically ran between 1300 and 1400 degrees Fahrenheit.

For the vast majority of the eighty men and women who took part in the ceremony, the experience was an exhilarating assertion of faith. Twelve people, however, were unsuccessful, and some were very badly burned. One man died. A frequently made observation at these walks seems particularly defiant of our Western reality. The long flowing togas that the walkers wear do not catch on fire, unless the believer has a lapse of faith. At that point, they spontaneously ignite.

Joseph Chilton Pearce tells how the English Society for Psychical Researchers in 1935 investigated two Indian fakirs. For weeks, the Indians did their firewalking routine while scientists from Oxford conducted various tests. The researchers concluded that, despite the seeming impossibility of the firewalk, neither deception nor illusion was involved. Perhaps the most exciting moment came when a scientist who had shown special fascination with the men's abilities was told by one of the fakirs that he, too, could walk the fire; he needed only to hold the fakir's hand. As Pearce says, "The good man was seized with faith that he could, shed his shoes, and hand-in-hand they walked the fire ecstatic and unharmed."

People who show little interest in scientific studies sometimes take a certain delight in placebo studies. The appeal stems from the irrefutability of the message they present. Humans have much greater power than they realize. Placebo studies suggest that positive expectations can create their own reality. In these studies patients are typically told that they are being given a pill to treat problems such as migraine headaches or depression. Unknown to the patients, the pills are inert sugar pills. The researchers then investigate to determine if patients experienced any effects from the "treatment."

A few examples:

> Dr. David Ayman gave placebos to subjects with hypertension. Not only did 82 percent of the patients show improvements; many even had side effects from the "medication." With placebos, the type of treatment is not of essence; the person's belief in the treatment is. In other experiments,

when mistletoe and extract from watermelons were given to hypertense patients, a significant number reported a reduction in their blood pressure.

In a study reported in the *World Journal of Surgery,* cancer patients were told they were receiving a new powerful type of chemotherapy. Thirty-one percent of the patients lost all their hair even though a placebo was being administered.

Dr. Marianne Frankenhauser gave women a placebo, but told them they were sleeping pills. The women reported feeling more tired and depressed than previously. There were corresponding physiological responses: Systolic and diastolic blood pressures lowered, and reaction times slowed. Later these same women were given identical pills, but this time they were told the pills were stimulants. They now reported feeling more alert and happy. Tangible measures also moved according to their beliefs about the pills. Blood pressure was higher, and reaction times were faster.

The power of the mind to influence warts has been known for many years. *The Healer Within,* by Steven Locke, M.D., and Douglas Colligan, tells of one unique way patients used their own inner resources, without knowing it, to vanquish their warts: "During the 1920s Dr. Bruno Bloch was a world-famous wart specialist in Zurich. The secret of his success was a 'wart-killing machine,' a wonderful apparatus that emitted an impressive noise, glittered with flashing lights, and—Bloch told his patients—beamed lethal antiwart rays at the offending growth. Patients were cured by the dozens. [In fact] the apparatus was a totally useless electronic creation with a motor inside that whirred and whirred and did little else. Somehow in the belief in Dr. Bloch's gadget the true medicine lay."

The influence of placebos has been demonstrated on a wide range of afflictions, including ulcers, acne, pain, and psychiatric disorders. They can even affect cancer, heart disease, multiple sclerosis, and diabetes.

By definition, placebos lack intrinsic value. They are a medium through which we channel our own innate power. They work where direct effort to enlist this power may fail because most people find it easier to believe in someone or something other than themselves. One woman, who did extraordinarily well with her advanced breast cancer, has some insight about the power she attributed to her various treatments. In her effort to overcome a terminal diagnosis, she was simultaneously involved in five different alternative approaches. She explains why: "I think I needed those therapies. I hung onto them and attributed to them a certain power that was in fact my own power, but I didn't have the confidence to stand up and claim it."

Whether Father DiOrio has invoked the power of God directly to intervene in healing or somehow catalyzed the "inner healer" (or, if one prefers, "the god within") may not really matter. In either case, he has demonstrated the essential human qualities of all gifted healers, the most significant being his concern with the well-being of the whole person. "Inner healing" is really his primary mission.

Father DiOrio forms an intense empathic relationship, however brief, with each person he attempts to heal. During the service, he says that he feels pain in different parts of his body. By directing his attention to these pains, he knows what maladies specific members of the congregation are suffering from. Like other powerful healers, he communicates confidence that the individual can get well, yet he never claims credit for successful outcomes. Over and over he states that he is not the source of the cure, merely the agent who happens to channel the curative forces. Father DiOrio believes that his capacity to embrace and care for another human being is essential. He says: "If I have full compassion, actually feel the core of a person's being, all of God's strength that's in me goes out of me and into that person. Then the healing takes place." Ultimately, then, his attempt to heal is an act of love.

BARBARA DAWSON

The five colors blind the eye.
The five tones deafen the ear.
The five flavors dull the taste.
Racing and hunting madden the mind.
Precious things lead one astray.

Therefore the sage is guided by what he feels and not by what he sees.
He lets go of that and chooses this.

Tao Te Ching, by Lao Tsu,
translated by Gia-Fu Feng
and Jane English

Barbara Dawson first felt a small hard lump in her breast more than eight years ago. She assumed it was nothing, and, unfortunately, when she mentioned it to her gynecologist, he also dismissed it. By the time the cancer was diagnosed two years later, it had spread with devastating consequences: She was expected to die shortly.

Barbara has seen many physicians since then. For this account, medical information was obtained from the first oncologist who treated her as well as the last. Although Barbara's condition is still considered medically unresolved, both oncologists indicated that she has done unusually well. There is considerable disagreement, however, when they attempt to quantify just how unusual the course of her illness has been. Barbara's original oncologist estimated the chances that she would still be alive today as 1 in 1,000; her last oncologist suggested the probability was 1 in 3. He was also asked to speculate why she did so well compared to other patients. Rather than acknowledging the possible value of her own efforts, his only response was, "biology of the disease."

Unlike any of the other extraordinary survivors interviewed for this book, Barbara Dawson was reticent to discuss her illness. In our initial phone conversation, I explained the nature of the project. Though our contact was warm and enjoyable, lasting well over an hour, she did not make a commitment to participate. She wanted time to think about it. Her reason for caution made it clear just how valuable her input would be. She explained: "To find the answers to the questions you are asking, I have to reach awfully deep, to touch and talk from my soul. Sometimes that's a scary place to be." She also wondered whether it was in her interest to spend so much time focusing on her life with cancer: "I don't want to be known as the person who had cancer. I want to break away from my identity with cancer and reclaim my wellness."

During our next conversation, she said that after giving it much thought, she would join me in "a process of mutual exploration." She felt that the process would further her own self-understanding, and, if her story could benefit others, she wanted to be of service.

Barbara was open, gentle, and reflective. Yet, when something struck her as funny, which was often, she would burst into hearty, almost raucous laughter. Once when I commented how wonderfully infectious her laugh was, she laughed again and told me that she had inherited it from her father.

She asked to know who I was. She listened in a very special way, and I shared some personal details of my life. Since we communicated only by phone and letter, I had no idea what she looked like, except that a colleague had told me she was fortyish, beautiful, and tall.

After about three months, once the initial interviewing was completed, we made plans to get together. A week before our scheduled meeting, however, Barbara called to cancel. She was starting a new job on that day. I asked if she would still be working with young children. She told me that she had decided to try something completely different. She was going to be the ombudsperson at a local health maintenance organization. Though Barbara had no formal training for this new line of work, the story she now shares demonstrates how well prepared she is to help work out complaints between patients and their doctors. Barbara began:

My own childhood wasn't that bad. I know people who had it much worse. But most of them had someone, a mother, a father, a relative, to help them deal. I didn't. So it seems that in my life nothing was dealt with.

My sister, two and a half years older than me, was sick with polio before I ever went to school. It was a dramatic illness. She recovered, but we were all quarantined, which meant that we were isolated from the outside world.

In my family, you were supposed to stand tall. But my older brother didn't "measure up." He was a whiny sort of child with a constant ache or pain. He was always symptomatic. I thought to myself, "Oh God, I never want to be like that!"

So I put up a very tough front even when I was in real pain, and I developed a false sense of myself. I never wanted anyone else to know how much I was hurting. I held on with a passion, afraid that if I let go, if I even admitted feeling weak or in pain, I'd be destroyed and I'd have nothing left.

I told my parents that I loved this man, an American, and I was going to leave England. They were totally against my coming to the United States, but I found myself taking off.

When I arrived here, I lost my identity. I was not American, and I was no longer English. I left my city to live in a small town. I was no longer my father's daughter. I didn't know who I was.

I came to the United States with the fantasy that the move would free me. My family had been very overprotective. My education was conservative and very rigid.

Suddenly I was trying to break free of all these restraints that I had been accustomed to. I was just overwhelmed. With all this freedom, I was fearful that somehow I would disgrace my family back home. My natural response was to shut myself down.

I was in awe of the liberation that I felt American women had. Comparatively, English women didn't seem at all autonomous. I was very curious. I wanted to be a part of it, but I also wanted what was familiar. I was in limbo, neither here nor there.

As a young child, I felt that I was destined to suffer greatly. It sounds really weird, but a part of me almost looked forward to it. It was the challenge in life for me. Of course, another part of me greatly feared it because I did not know what form it was going to take.

In my day-to-day life, there was a lot of suffering. My religious upbringing had a lot to do with my keeping myself in a suffering mode. That's what life was supposed to be. Suffering gave life meaning. It sounds crazy and weird, and I wish it had not been like that, but when I really wanted to feel good about myself, suffering was the thing to do.

Half of me felt that the religious stuff was just foolishness, and I did not want any part of it. And the other half of me was so drawn to it. I felt so good, so worthy, so righteous. It was very compelling. There were these two very distinct halves—and probably more. These opposing sides were gnawing on me, creating ambivalence and guilt. I had mixed feelings constantly, and I could not come to terms with them.

Guilt was so overwhelming that I did not understand how I could continue living unless I found a way to suffer greatly. If I didn't suffer, I would have to find a way to let the world know that I was a bad person. I needed to repent. I was so bad that I did not deserve to continue living without some sort of suffering in my life. To me, there was no forgiveness.

All these feelings, all of this ambivalence, created a tremendous amount of stress. It finally affected me physically.

Once I had the cancer, I felt almost relieved. "It's OK. You've suffered enough. Now you can do something positive for yourself."

It was as if I had brought the illness upon myself, and I was the only one who could undo it. But I never imagined I would do something so serious to myself. I thought, "Oh my goodness, how am I ever going to undo this?"

I had recognized a lump in my breast for a long time. I would mention it to my gynecologist, but he never seemed that concerned about it. He thought I was too young to have anything like cancer.

I was sure it was nothing, until periodically my breast started to get very painful. I decided to go to a surgeon. He said it was a lump that needed to be aspirated. I knew that he was wrong because it was just too hard to be aspirated. He tried to aspirate it.

I felt so healthy. It was very difficult to believe what I was hearing. I never felt sick.

When the doctor first said "cancer," when he used the word, I suddenly felt unworthy. Cancer was a bad word. It wasn't like "stroke" or "Parkinson's" or "diabetes." I felt that people were not going to want to be around me.

My husband's reaction that afternoon was incredible. We were sitting in the doctor's office together. My doctor said, "You know, there is no way this can be overcome, but we can do this and this and this to postpone things."

My husband said, "Well, have you ever seen anybody overcome this before?"

The doctor said, "No, I haven't."

My husband automatically turned to me and said, "Well, Barbara here is the first person!"

I was sitting there in shock. Oh my God. I had no idea what I was supposed to do. But he said it, and I'll never forget that moment.

If he hadn't said something like that, I don't know what would have happened. I needed him to have that faith. I needed someone to believe more strongly in me than I could.

That was the first time I understood the confidence he had in me. I felt incredibly empowered by it. Empowered.

I knew that I had to figure out for myself what to do.

I went to get other opinions, but they all said the same thing: "Yes, you have cancer." Point-blank they told me, "You probably have only a year."

The first surgeon wanted to do a mastectomy immediately. I then went to a second surgeon, who brought in the oncologist. The oncologist said, "No, we need to do more testing first." They did the bone scan and found it had spread to my bones, to my spine. With this, the mastectomy was unnecessary.

When they agreed that my ovaries needed to be removed, my body felt like it was being attacked. I was very threatened, and yet there seemed to be no choice. Everyone was putting pressure on me to act very quickly. The doctors felt that I was just denying and delaying things and that I had to do something very quickly. I believed, and my husband believed—because we were so overwhelmed—that I needed to do something immediately.

I went to Rochester and saw two or three more doctors. They confirmed what the others had said. Then I came home and went to my GP. If I wanted, he would give me the names of some other doctors in New York City or Boston, or wherever I wanted to go, but he didn't see the point.

I was afraid to go someplace else. My illness was already being handled in such an impersonal way. I did not want to go to someplace even bigger where I imagined standing in a long line waiting to see yet another doctor whom I had never met before to discuss the most intimate of details about my body and my life.

Besides, it seemed that these doctors just handed information on to each other. I didn't feel that these doctors would speak for themselves. Once a doctor had my records, I didn't think he was really willing to question another doctor's diagnosis. I don't have any hard evidence of this, but it was always my feeling.

At the time, I was teaching in a long-term substitute position. I went in to talk with the principal and let him know what was going on. I said I was going to take a week off before Christmas vacation because I had to have a hysterectomy.

He said, "Well, don't bother coming back."

That was like telling me, "Go ahead and die, lady." I felt so bad. I wanted to say, "You don't understand, this is what is going to make me well. I have to be with these children."

I felt like a leper. It seemed nobody could understand what the feeling was. I was being pushed out of society into a small segment of people called "those who have cancer."

When I really needed somebody who would have faith in me, no matter how bad the odds were, there was no one. My husband couldn't maintain his initial conviction with no support from the environment. I was abandoned by mankind; everybody had left me to die.

I told the principal, "I have a contract. I'm going to finish out the year."

I was searching for a person who could give me some hope, because it was so hard by myself. I needed to be reassured by somebody else that the remotest possibility existed that I could possibly get well.

One of the doctors I went to see was a radiologist. His specialty was reading X-rays.

He said, "Well, it looks 90 percent sure that it has metastasized to the bones."

When I said, "Can you be 100 percent sure?" He said, "No, there certainly are hot spots, but I can't really tell you 100 percent." I think he felt confident enough in his specialty to say something a little different from the others. He said that the only way to be 100 percent certain was to have a bone biopsy. He said the procedure was very painful and that getting the bone marrow out without contamination was difficult. He did not encourage me to go through that.

His opinion was the only one I really listened to because it seemed the most hopeful. According to everyone else, I was doomed.

I agreed to an oophorectomy [removal of the ovaries]. But because I never felt sick, part of me always questioned whether the diagnosis was true. I mean, I was jogging the morning I went in for surgery. In some ways I felt, OK, I'll let you do this to me now, but I'll show you. I'm going to come back. I'm going to regain my sense of dignity and self-worth. I felt they were trying to take that away from me.

After the surgery, I was in a lot of pain and discomfort. I had lost weight, and it took a while to get my strength back.

The week I was in the hospital, my husband had a client come in whose sister had just died of cancer. He gave my husband a Bernie Siegel tape for me to listen to. It spoke directly to my experience; I felt legitimized. I found him one of the few doctors who doesn't want to take away their patients' power.

I have a friend who's a doctor. He would visit me in the hospital and want to know how I was doing. Over time, I realized he was very afraid of my illness, afraid that I would die. I didn't expect it, and it seems surprising, but doctors are as afraid of death as anybody else.

Now I understand that when I get medical advice and they put pressure on me to act quickly, I have to figure out how much of it is based on legitimate concerns and how much is based on their fears.

After my surgery, I said to my friend that I didn't care what his fears were or what my doctors' fears were. No one was ever going to get me to respond that quickly again. I probably would have made different decisions if I had allowed myself to take the time, but I think I was too afraid to wait.

Right after the surgery, I went back to teaching. I knew that I needed to be with those children. They were the only people in my life I felt I could really be myself with. They're so uninhibited; I felt that I could be uninhibited with them. With adults, I needed to be this other person who really did not seem like me.

The children gave something to me that I really needed. I had to let them do that, and they would. There was magic and beauty in being with them. They were wonderful, and I think they really benefited from the experience as well.

There were times when I might be writing on the blackboard or listening to a child, and I would think, "Oh my God. I must be terribly sick. What am I doing here?" I would feel tremendous strain, lower-back pain, and it would seem like my whole back was going to give out. I had been told that the cancer was in my spine.

To get through those times, I had to get into a different conscious-ness, to tap into the positive, to believe that there was a good possibility that I wasn't a sick person. Over and over, I would say to myself, "I am OK. Look what I'm doing, I'm standing here teaching. I couldn't be that sick."

Trying to uphold this attitude for myself wasn't always easy. But trying to make others feel OK was much more of a burden. I looked weaker, I had lost weight, and people were, of course, overwhelmed by the diagnosis. Somehow I had to present myself to others as though I was all right. "No, really, I'm OK" over and over again. People seemed afraid that I was going to die on them.

At the end of the school year, I applied for the same teaching position and didn't get it.

My whole life, I felt like I was trying to prove myself. Here I am, supposed to die, and I still have to prove myself. It seemed that I had to prove to people that I could continue living. It made me very angry.

That summer, I knew I had to go away. I couldn't stand it anymore. My husband and I were just too close. Everything was up for grabs, including the relationship. I questioned if I needed to break away from him. So it was a very scary time. Fortunately my husband could give me the space I needed. I'm sure he needed time to himself. He would support any decision that I had to make.

It was time to stand on my own two feet. I would welcome support and guidance, but the initiative had to be mine.

I had gone through life playing a guessing game. "What does this person want me to say? What does that person want me to do?" I was always trying to please someone else. I had gotten very good at figuring out what would please others, but I really didn't know what I wanted.

Suddenly I didn't have to worry about being overly good or overly this or overly anything. I was going to die. The time limit on my life made me feel much better about doing exactly what I wanted.

I would decide what I needed and then just do it.

I knew what I had to do. I didn't hem and haw. I didn't wonder if I had enough money. I didn't wonder who was going to come with me. For the first time, none of those things mattered. I knew things would fall into place once I took the initiative and made the decision.

I felt like a leper when I left my home to spend the summer at the Options Institute.* People were afraid of me, and I was afraid to be around people. They didn't want to talk about cancer, such a dreaded thing. People seemed fearful they could catch it from me. I felt very alone.

The first night, we sat around a circle, each one of us telling something about who we were. My reason for being there, I said, was because I had cancer, and I did not know if I was going to live or die.

Barry Neil Kaufman, the codirector of the Institute, said to me, "You know, it doesn't really matter whether you live or die."

It was such a relief to hear him say that. All of a sudden, he had given me permission not to live. I didn't have to prove myself, by living, to anybody.

But they also believed in miracles. I really needed people who could verbalize that kind of support. They believed that love could help people get well.

The Institute grounds were beautiful. My frame of mind was so peaceful. I was in some heavenly type of place. Every once in a while, they would try and bring you down to earth, but I was flying. I mean, I went to see Bernie Siegel while I was there and that was the most grounding thing I did. [Barbara laughed.]

A strong sense of community, of family, developed. This was

*The Options Institute, located in Sheffield, Massachusetts, offers counseling workshops designed to enhance personal development.

probably the first time I felt really accepted in a group of people. I was freed up.

When the Options Institute summer session ended, my plan was to begin their mentorship program. I would go down there once every three weeks. On the first morning, I left my house at 5:30 A.M. to get there in time. It was very foggy. I was concentrating for such a long time, trying to see through the fog, that I guess I was mesmerized by the road. When I drove off the road, I was so startled that instead of putting my foot on the brake, I put it on the accelerator. I started going very fast. Fortunately, there was a field in front of me; unfortunately there was a tree in it. I totaled my car.

The Options process helped me to listen to myself more. I was seeing things as signs. I interpreted the accident as an indication I was going in the wrong direction. So I stopped going down there.

I became very interested in magic. I went to a workshop on the Healing Power of Laughter and Play by Joel Goodman. He does humor and laughter and magic tricks. I started doing magic with my nieces, and they loved it. People would come in, and I would do magic tricks, and everybody was so wonderful, they just let me do it. Learning magic was important. It wasn't something that just happened, that you didn't have any control over. You do have control, and you can make magic. You just don't let everybody know how you do it. [She laughed again.]

Up to this point, I was seeing my oncologist regularly. I wanted him to listen to the tape that I had from Bernie Siegel. He kept telling me that he didn't have a tape recorder at work. The more I talked like this, the more it disturbed him. He thought I was right off the wall. He seemed wary of me even though the cancer was not growing nearly as fast as he thought it would. But rather than being delighted for me, he seemed upset by it.

It was very upsetting for me to go to see the doctor. I wanted to talk with somebody who was in a powerful position in regard to my health who was invested in whatever might work. I wanted to share with them the things that I was doing. Instead, I felt like I was fighting the authorities. I never felt they were really on my side or that they wanted to work with me. I was this woman that they had to put up with. I think that's when I decided that I needed alternatives.

I started going to Kripalu.* I would see their homeopathic physician and attend their seminars. I was also seeing a chiropractor. My regular doctors thought I should be taking this medication called Tamoxifen. I refused, but I was fearful, wondering whether or not I was doing the right thing. Then my homeopathic doctor said perhaps I should take the Tamoxifen. That really threw me; he wasn't supposed to say that.

One afternoon, I was at my desk writing a paper. I had begun a part-time master's program in counseling. I was sitting there touching my neck when I felt some nodes. The doctors had told me that if the cancer spread, it probably would go upward, up to my neck. The glands were swollen. I was in danger. I became very preoccupied with the possibility that the cancer was spreading.

I called my chiropractor. He had once told me that if I ever needed anything more than what he could give me, he would try to find people who could help me out.

I had trust in him. I knew he wanted to do something to help me, and he made me feel very taken care of.

It's not legal, but I had no reservations when he gave me the name and number of the Manner's Clinic, in Mexico. My mind was set on the right track because I felt my chiropractor would only recommend something that would benefit me. I talked to doctors at the clinic to get as much information as I could.

I called Dr. Harold Manner right at his home in Tijuana, Mexico. I made plans to leave on the ninth of November. I told him my birthday was on the tenth.

He said, "That's perfect. We'll celebrate your birthday."

Everything I did down there revolved around the theme of rebirthing.

During this time, and for the next year, I was constantly regressing into a childlike state. I needed to grow up all over again, but this time, the way I wanted to.

I needed to regress to those early years filled with magic and fantasy. I truly believe that one of the key secrets of doing well with a major illness is to return to the childlike belief that anything is possible. But it is very difficult for most adults to do that.

---

*Kripalu is a spiritual retreat center with a wide range of programs; yoga, body work, nutrition, health and fitness. It is located in Lenox, Massachusetts.

Psychologically, the treatment in Mexico felt incredibly life-supporting. Unlike chemotherapy, the treatment was presented as something that would enhance my immune system. Basically the treatment would cleanse out my whole system and then feed it with these nutrients. For eighteen days, I received an intravenous solution. The theory was that the substance would break down the tumor, and simultaneously they would be flushing out any floating debris.

For the year prior to this treatment, I had been working very hard on meditation and self-hypnosis. I could get myself into a very relaxed state. While taking in the solution, I think I was in some hypnotic trance, or maybe it was a psychotic trance. [Barbara laughed.] They were putting a magic solution into my veins that was going to make me well.

Last year, I went through radiation treatment. I wanted my doctor to say to me, once the treatment was completed, that he would put me in the hospital and feed me vitamin C or other nutrients to enhance my immune system. I think I was afraid to request it because I know how little regard is given to nutrition. But I was very disappointed and angry that it never occurred to him to do that.

When I first started seeing this latest oncologist, he was very belligerent. He thought I was a crazy woman.

He constantly tells me that somehow I am different. My cancer is not responding like anybody else's he has seen. It's a very slow-growing kind of cancer—so far. He makes sure to tell me this all the time. I don't appreciate it.

He says, "You've got to take this. There's nothing else that works, you're just into denial." I feel like he's angry with me. He frightens me quite a bit. Every time I go there, he says, "Are you ready to take the Tamoxifen now?" And I say, "No."

I know that when I leave there, he's not feeling that great. He wants to give me something. When he can't give me something, I think it makes him feel helpless. I feel like I'm doing something bad to him. It's an awful feeling.

Every once in a while I say to myself, "I'm never going back to see him." But then I laugh and say, "Well, maybe this man will finally learn something from this."

[The interviews with Barbara went on for three months. During this time, she had an appointment with her oncologist. She described the visit:]

Our discussions here brought some things to life. I realized how angry I was with him. On this last visit, I said, "I'd like to talk with you. Could we sit down?" I said, "I don't appreciate your attitude. By keeping everything in such a negative light, it's very hard for me to maintain my good feelings."

Without any real discussion, he immediately said, "I know, I know. You want to see somebody else. Right? Who do you want to see?"

But I did not necessarily want to see somebody else. I was trying to see if we couldn't negotiate the relationship, if we couldn't make things better for both of us.

To him, I was a complainer. I was a patient who wasn't fitting into the mold. He was very happy to hand me over to somebody else.

He misunderstood me, the way I talk. When I have something to say, I get very emotional. There's a lot of force behind it. I think the other person usually feels something, even if he's not used to feeling anything.

I was really saying to him, I'm sorry, but I can no longer let you treat me only like a disease. Either you have to treat me like a person or I have to leave. I think he answered that he was not willing to treat me like a person. I was either a disease or nothing.

I did make an appointment with another doctor, but I'm having reservations. I really don't know whether I can go through this again. I want to give up on them. I feel frustrated, I feel like I'm having to put much more energy into the relationship than they are willing to. I feel very disappointed.

Radiation and chemotherapy have always felt like something imposed on me, shoved down my throat. When something is presented like that, I resist it automatically. My body just says, "Whoa, slow down."

Reading about Jill Ireland's story was helpful.

While pregnant, she was in a minor car accident. She was thrown up against the dash, and her knees were shoved into her abdomen.

She went to see a physician because there was some bleeding. The physician said she was fine.

But soon she went into labor. Her husband, Charles Bronson, left the room to get a doctor. She started to bleed. Her mother went to get a towel. Alone in her room, she squatted on the floor and gave birth to a child who was born dead. She describes vividly what it was like to find herself with this dead infant in a pool of blood.

She describes the loss of her breast; they removed her breast because of cancer. She wonders what they did with the breast. Did they just throw it away? She wonders what they did with the baby that she never saw again. Did they just throw him away?

She loses a piece of her body and practically nobody acknowledges it. What did they do with it? Just put it in a garbage bag? Did they put it in an incinerator? I mean, all your body parts are important, and they just slice it off. It gives you an image of how brutal the whole procedure can be. People who have lost a part of their body, part of themself, have a tremendous amount to deal with.

Hospital personnel don't deal with it. In medical school, doctors are trained to deal with human body parts in such an objective, sometimes disrespectful, manner. I remember talking to a physician at the Options Institute. He told me how they had to go to the lab and do dissections. There were these great big vats with human body parts floating in formaldehyde. Interns would have to reach in and pick out the human body parts that they were going to dissect. They were desensitizing the students to the fact that they were dealing with the bodies of human beings. It's little wonder that doctors treat people the way they do.

When you learn you have a serious illness, I think it's important to find people who have been through it themselves, who have passed through some of the critical moments and know what it's like. Or else you need someone who has worked with others who have been through it.

You can join a support group, even if you don't want to be an active member. It can be helpful just to hear what others have to say. When you have cancer, there is a tendency to withdraw, to close up. At first there may be a desire to latch onto something because of panic, but then you may find yourself withdrawing. It may seem that others around you are supporting the sense of hopelessness. But I don't think that they are. People who are closest to you are desperately struggling with their own fears.

Ideally you will find someone—a counselor, a therapist, a friend— who can help you listen to yourself. Because, if you listen—really listen—to yourself, you may get a sense of what you can do to make yourself healthier. But when you're fearful, you can't listen. When you're fearful, you can't relax, you can't be by yourself, you can't be quiet, you can't let go. Meditation can help you relax so you can feel more assured that you're hearing your true self.

For some people who are very ill, there is nothing to do. Their bodies may be telling them that they really are at a final stage, that they are at a point where they can't recoup their physical resources.

I think meditation and imagery are the key to this inner knowing. Like everything else I did, I read about different kinds of imagery and adapted something that seemed right for me. I found this tape that sounded like a waterfall. Every day after school, I would come home and envision my body as healthy. I would sit very still, listen to the tape, and imagine that this waterfall was cleansing my system. I used the information my doctors gave to me as the opening image. Then I would picture the cancer being healed. My body was being cleansed of the cancer; I was healing my body.

The more I visualized, the more powerful the technique became. It's not something you can just do one time and have it work. You have to practice to get better at it. It takes effort and persistence and real belief that it could possibly work. It's not like taking a pill— "Here, take this. It will make you feel better." It requires a lot of self-motivation.

I did not know if it was going to work or how. I did not want to share it with other people because I knew they would think it strange and just so much hocus-pocus. I felt no need to convince anyone else. And I never wanted to impose it on anyone else with cancer. Because if someone with cancer isn't ready, if the timing isn't right, if they are not ready to take charge, you will only burden them.

The imagery, like my own decisions, felt very right, no matter how weird it may have seemed to anybody else. I also did not know what else to do. It seemed like the right thing to do. Of course, there would be times of questioning.

OBSERVATIONS

Barbara Dawson had waited for most of her life to get cancer, or something equally devastating. In fact, she told us that the cancer diagnosis brought some relief. She no longer had to live with the constant anxiety that something awful was about to happen—the worst had already happened.

Finally there was consistency with what she felt she deserved and her objective reality. Bernie Siegel, the healer who Barbara herself said often seemed to express what she was feeling, has commented that the suffering associated with devastating illness can act like a crucifixion, sowing the seeds of salvation. He said, "So many people have been unloved, used and blamed, and the disease can awaken them. Disease releases the guilt that punishes individuals for all their sins. Then they can go on and be who they really want to be."

Cancer cleared the slate for Barbara; she had paid for her sins and was free to be herself. Her effort to survive could have been a rerun of old ways, going through the motions of life, attempting to stay alive because she thought that's what was expected of her. But after the diagnosis, Barbara stopped trying so hard to please others. Ultimately she even gave herself permission to die—without feeling shame, without feeling that she had failed someone else. Free to die, she recognized that her true desire was to live, and, thus unconflicted, she could focus all of her considerable resources in the quest for life.

Barbara's personal power evolved through her struggle with cancer. While growing up, she was constantly fighting with herself. Since so much of her energy was consumed in these internal battles, she had little left to create her world. The language she chose to describe her life as a young adult reflected her feelings of disempowerment. For example, coming to the United States was a major life change, yet she described herself as passive: "I found myself taking off." It is as though her actions were not under her control.

My present sense of Barbara—a courageous, strong-willed, and quietly powerful woman—contrasts sharply with this earlier image, for there is no question that Barbara is now in charge of herself. To describe her decision-making process, she said, "I would decide what I needed, and then just do it. I knew what I had to do, I didn't hem and haw." Consider her most recent medical appointment, where she sat her doctor down and told him, "I don't appreciate your attitude."

In *The Crack in the Cosmic Egg,* Joseph Chilton Pearce states how enervating internal conflict can be:

> A mind divided by choices, confused by alternatives, is a mind robbed of power. The body reflects this. The ambiguous person is a machine out of phase, working against itself and tearing itself up. That person is an engine with sand in its crankcase, broken piston rods, water in its fuel lines. In spite of great effort and noise, nothing much happens.

Barbara herself believed that this internal conflict was at least one component of her cancer development.

The structure of cancer cells does not have the orderliness found with normal cells and may be so disorganized that it becomes impossible to identify their source of origin. Barbara thinks of her illness in metaphorical terms, suggesting that, at a cellular level, the disease was a microcosm of her life. She consistently describes her actions as disorganized and unfocused: "I didn't know who I was," "I was neither here nor there," "I was not an American and I was no longer English." Once she became ill, however, she approached life with more certainty. Whether she was planning a trip to Mexico or speaking with the school principal about her contract, she acted more decisively, trusting that her decisions were the right ones. Her purposefulness was especially apparent in the way she now approached conflict. During one interview, she spoke about the open disagreements with her doctors: "In the past, I always had internal conflicts, so I was a passive-aggressive kind of a fighter. I think perhaps the present conflict is good because I am fighting in a more open way than I ever had." She suggested that her internal state mirrors her external state and assumed that finding some peace in her life had benefits at a cellular level.

Barbara, like other survivors, felt that belief in recovery was critical. In order to believe, she had to return to a childlike state where anything was possible, including miracles. She nurtured her inner child, making certain she had plenty of room to play. Because Barbara's adult world seemed incapable of believing that a positive outcome was possible, she spent much time in the world of young children, where the boundaries separating fantasy and reality are fluid. Since young children are not so steeped in the nature of human limitations, the miraculous becomes commonplace, and the stage is set for the unexpected. *Why Me?* tells the story of Garrett Porter, a nine-year-old who successfully battled an inoperable brain tumor. He believed that his "childish" perspective was an important factor in his remarkable healing: "I went in there with an open mind. I was curious. I think that's what being a kid can do for you because adults have this false sense of reality—that maybe it's not possible."

Barbara had to go to extraordinary lengths to find a doctor who would not extinguish all hope. She wasn't seeking false promises, only an expert who would humbly grant that medical science did not know enough about the essence of life to make irrevocable pronouncements of doom. Less than a generation ago, physicians customarily did not tell their patients they had cancer. Today's swing toward full disclosure, however positive, does not necessarily mean that patients are getting the full picture. For, regardless of the statistical likelihood of recovery, there is always reason for hope; and the way a physician communicates the diagnosis is a medical intervention of great importance. Doctors who tell their patients, people who are especially vulnerable because of the crises in their lives, how much time they have left may be creating self-fulfilling prophecies. As Bernie Siegel said in an interview, "In some cases, physicians are literally killing people with words. I don't mean malpracticing, but I mean by taking away hope, predicting when they're going to die. Most people don't have the strength to cast off the death sentence, so they go home and die faster."

Barbara was not predisposed to seek alternative healing methods, but since she felt badly treated by the medical establishment, she began to look elsewhere for answers. She did not trust what her doctors told her because she felt uncared for and so found it necessary to get a second, third, and fourth medical opinion. She questioned whether or not the corroborating doctors were speaking for themselves or sheepishly supporting the opinion of a colleague. Her doubts are not paranoid. Physicians, like other professionals, do sometimes rubber-stamp their colleagues' opinions rather than risk disagreement. As one physician acknowledged in *How Can I Help?*:

> Even now, after years of experience, I'm very reluctant to challenge a colleague on a tricky diagnosis. It's a kind of dirty little secret in the medical profession. Everyone has a lot at

stake. We all cling to our authority and persona. It becomes a sort of unwritten code among physicians, the license to do that. Very delicate stuff. And who pays, by the way?

Barbara did not want to—or perhaps she could not—work with doctors who weren't respectful of her. Many of us have had the experience of trying to learn from a teacher who was technically competent but interpersonally deficient. In this situation, the acquisition of knowledge is slow and painful. Similarly employees do not perform up to capacity when they are working with a boss who is disrespectful and negative. Healing is certainly no less intimate a process. A doctor is not merely a dispenser and synthesizer of scientific knowledge, nor is a patient an inert receptacle. As Norman Cousins says, "Ultimately, it is the physician's respect for the human soul that determines the worth of his science."

There was no hope of deep intimacy in Barbara's life until she could reveal who she was. But, like most of us, she felt that certain parts of her being were too loathsome to share. Barbara wanted, most of all, to hide her pain and weakness: "I'd be destroyed and I'd have nothing left if these feelings were exposed." But since pain is a sacred part of who one is, cutting this off kept her a perpetual stranger. She dared not acknowledge her pain, even to herself. Until the cancer, she was disconnected from herself and driven to remain out of touch, for connecting with these feelings was the emotional equivalent of self-annihilation.

Lawrence LeShan believes that these feelings of hopeless isolation are common among people who contract cancer. He states that many patients "specifically expressed the idea that for years they had felt there was no way out of the emotional box they found themselves in short of death itself. . . . They feel that they can be themselves—and therefore unloved and alone—or that they can get rid of themselves to be someone else and thus be loved." The individual feels powerless to take any positive action, for all action is equally useless.

Barbara, however, pierced through this isolation. She found people at Kripalu and at the Options Institute with whom it seemed safe to take a chance and reveal who she was. As she herself came to recognize and accept her many different sides, she would insist that special others, such as her doctor, also acknowledge her wholeness.

After the diagnosis, Barbara was emotionally prepared to develop closer relationships than previously, but the circumstances also made it more difficult. People responded differently to her because she had cancer. Unfortunately her experience is a common one for the cancer patient. For example, in one study specifically concerned with the social support available to women with breast cancer, 72 percent of the patients said that they were treated differently once others knew they had cancer. One-half reported that they were avoided or feared.

The following excerpt from *Side Effects,* a Woody Allen book of short stories, captures many of our core fears. Meyer Iskowitz is in the hospital with cancer, and his poker buddy Lenny Mendel has finally come to visit him:

"How's it going, Meyer?" Mendel said weakly as he tried to maintain a respectable distance from the bed.

"Who's that? Mendel? Is that you, Lenny?"

"I been busy. Otherwise I'd have come sooner."

"Oh it's so nice of you to bother. I'm so glad to see you."

"How are you, Meyer?"

"How am I? I'm going to beat this thing, Lenny. Mark my words. I'm going to beat this thing."

"Sure you will, Meyer," Lenny Mendel said in a feeble voice, constricted by tension. "In six months you'll be back cheating at cards. Ha, ha, no seriously, you never cheated."

Keep it light, Mendel thought, keep the one liners coming. Treat him like he isn't dying, Mendel thought, recalling advice he had read on the subject. In the stuffy little room, Mendel imagined he was inhaling billows of the virulent cancer germs as they emanated from Iskowitz and multiplied in the warm air. "I bought you a *Post,*" Lenny said, laying the offering down on the table.

"Sit, sit. Where you running? You just came," Meyer said warmly.

"I'm not running. It's just that the visiting instructions say to keep the visits short for the comfort of the patients."

"So what's new?" Meyer asked.

Resigned to chat the full time till eight [ten minutes], Mendel pulled up a chair (not too close) and tried to make conversation about cards, sports, headlines, and finances, always awkwardly conscious of the overriding, horrible fact that, despite Iskowitz's optimism, he would never be leaving this hospital alive. Mendel was perspiring and felt woozy. The pressure, the forced gaiety, the pervasiveness of disease and awareness of his own fragile mortality caused his neck to grow stiff and his mouth to dry up. He wanted to leave. It was already five after eight and he hadn't been asked to go. The visiting rules were lax. He squirmed in his seat as Iskowitz spoke softly of the old days and after five more depressing minutes Mendel thought he would faint.

Like many people with cancer, Barbara experienced intense feelings of isolation; she had been "abandoned by mankind." Disconnectedness of such magnitude threatens survival because it can shrivel a person's will to live. The way out of this box begins when either patient or "visitor" expresses what he or she is feeling. When we admit our fear, anger, or sadness, barriers that obstruct our loving feelings start to fall.

Through meditation, Barbara calmed herself, focused her concentration, and helped intuit the course of action that would serve her best. By quieting her mind, she was able to tap the power of the unconscious and listen to the wisdom of her inner healer. The internal chatter of the mind is constant. Meditation is a technique to quiet this chatter, to tame the wildness of the mind. The more we learn to be still, the more control we have over the mind's vast powers. For those unfamiliar with it, meditation can appear an exotic or alien process. Ironically, once meditation techniques are described, they sometimes seem too simple to be of service.

I believe that meditation is the most important commitment a person, sick or well, can make to improve the quality of life. Although some people have incredible beginning experiences, practice is necessary. The range of meditation possibilities is great. In *Journey of Awakening,* Ram Dass offers a guidebook to meditators, while Harvard cardiologist Herbert Benson provides a more "scientific" approach in *The Relaxation Response.*

Barbara had her own theory about why she got cancer: She felt that her constant state of ambivalence as well as her need to suffer were causative. She did not judge or blame herself for the past but used these insights as a roadmap telling her what changes needed to be made. Barbara obviously found it helpful to make connections between her past behavior and her disease. This does not mean, however, that it would have been helpful if someone else had foisted this interpretation upon her. People with serious illness don't want or need someone else suggesting that they created their illness, nor do they want to be told that they can take control of their lives if only they choose to. Asking a sick person why he gave himself an illness is simplistic. And it almost always feels that the person who asks is also passing judgment. Such statements may make the healthy person feel better, but they rarely reflect the compassion that the patient needs.

In fact, as more and more individuals feel responsible for their health, some will overdo it. Although everyone can be encouraged to realize the full range of their power, some people may need help coming to terms with their human limitations.

When someone is ill, the most valued gift we can give is rarely tangible and seldom is it advice, no matter how good our intentions. Treya Killam Wilber, a counselor who had breast cancer, wrote in the *Journal of Transpersonal Psychology* about "What Kind of Help Really Helps." She says that now when she is with someone who is ill, she works to remember that

> Listening is helping. Listening is giving. I try to be emotionally accessible to them, to reach through my own fears and touch them, to maintain human contact. I find there are many fearful things we can laugh at together once we've allowed ourselves to be truly afraid. I try to steer clear of the temptation to define imperatives for others, even imperatives such as fight for your life, change yourself, or die consciously. I try not to push people to move in directions I have chosen or think I might choose for myself. I try to stay in touch with my own fear that I might one day find myself in the same situation they are in.

Listening to someone else's pain and confusion, while knowing there may be nothing we can do to lessen their suffering, is a gift from the heart.

RELATED RESEARCH

When Barbara Dawson left England to live in the United States, she found herself isolated from all that was familiar. Although general research findings don't necessarily have any relevance for the individual, there is some evidence that suggests social isolation poses an increased risk of cancer for women. In 1965, two epidemiologists, Peggy Reynolds and George Kaplan, gave questionnaires to 6,928 adults, none of whom had a previous history of cancer. Seventeen years later, nearly 500 people in this group had developed cancer. The findings were presented to the Society of Behavioral Medicine. Women who were initially identified as socially isolated (those with few close human relationships and those who felt alone even when in the company of others) were twice as likely to have contracted cancer and three times as likely to have died from cancer when compared with woman who had many social contacts and did not feel socially isolated.

Barbara sought multiple medical opinions before agreeing to a course of action, and even then felt she acted precipitously. Although the ideal mind-set is faith in one's doctors and treatment once a decision is made, there is evidence that a certain amount of vigilance is called for. Researchers from the Rand Corporation and the University of California, Los Angeles, investigated the medical records of 386 patients who had heart-bypass operations. The results, published in the *Journal of the American Medical Association,* found that 14 percent of the operations were "inappropriate," and an additional 30 percent were questionable. In one of the hospitals studied, only 37 percent of the coronary bypass operations were considered appropriate. Extrapolated from this study, a conservative estimate finds that every year, 40,000 people risk their lives by having an operation that is dangerous, costly, and inappropriate.

Even more disconcerting was a study published in the *Annals of Internal Medicine* in October 1988. The records of 182 patients were reviewed by a team of three physicians. The cases came from twelve hospitals, and the patients had died while they were being treated for pneumonia, heart ailments, and strokes. The conclusions: All three physicians who reviewed the cases agreed that 14 percent of the deaths probably should have been prevented, and two of three physicians agreed that 27 percent of the deaths were probably preventable. Doctors' mistakes that led to their patients' deaths included prescribing the wrong medication for pneumonia, misdiagnosing strokes because blood cultures or spinal taps weren't administered, and improper treatment of patients with chest pains.

There was a hollow ring to the research team leader's attempts to allay the fears of prospective patients by highlighting what was apparently the statistical good news: Any given individual going into the hospital would probably not be killed by a medical mistake. He said: "The overwhelming majority, over 95 percent, of the people admitted to a hospital don't die. This is a nonissue for them. So it's important to put this in perspective. Of the one-quarter to one-sixth of the 5 percent who do die, their death was probably preventable."

CAROLE MATTHEWS AND BETTY PRESTON

The fear of death is the basic fear that influences all others, a fear from which no one is immune no matter how disguised it may be.

The Denial of Death, Ernest Becker

The two women who tell their stories in this chapter present themselves very differently. Betty Preston is elderly, effusive, and affectionate. Carole Matthews, only about half Betty's age, interacts much more carefully. Betty is blond and full-figured, and reminds me of the grandmother I always wished for while growing up. Carole is dark, thin, and exotically attractive.

Despite their differences in presentation, the women share an experience that has had the most profound impact on each of them. Both spent time on that fine line between life and death; one may have actually crossed over for a brief visit. Their encounters with death have left them forever changed.

Carole Matthews

When we first met, Carole Matthews had been dealing with a lethal malignancy for four years. And, although her course of illness was going unusually well, she was not especially hopeful about her chances of survival. She equivocated, at times believing that a miracle was possible, but generally she expressed far less optimism than any of the other survivors.

As we approached the end of the interview, Carole said there was something more she needed to say. Her embarrassment was palpable, and she voiced concern that her revelation could sound bizarre. But the belief that her offering might help others enabled her to discuss the details of an intimate daily ritual.

The visualization process she then shared with me was actually quite similar to the techniques now used by many people. In order to understand the significance of her experience, however, it is necessary to put her practice of visualization in perspective. She began using visualization ten years ago. At that time, scarcely a handful of practitioners were familiar with it. Carole possesses a raw wisdom, but she was not formally educated and certainly not versed in "New Age" thinking. She never learned about visualization from someone else. The idea that it could be healing, and the decision to make it part of her regular treatment, sprang from someplace deep within her.

The interview with Carole was conducted about five years ago. She was thirty-eight years old and lived with her husband and two sons. We spoke in her doctor's office, located in the radiation oncology department of a city hospital. She smoked intermittently throughout the interview.

Carole's original diagnosis was inoperable, undifferentiated lung cancer, with a particularly aggressive cell type. Her oncologist reported that when the cancer was first discovered, he felt that the chances were only 1 in 100 that she could survive for five years. To follow up on Carole's progress, I contacted this oncologist again (nine years after the diagnosis). When I inquired how she was doing, he responded, "Believe it or not, she's alive and well." Then he told me that a few months ago he had been asked to complete some Social Security disability forms recertifying her terminal status. He knew she needed the money, but he couldn't do it in good conscience. He explained that there was just no way she could still be considered terminal.

In my interview with her, she spoke of her actions when she first learned she had cancer:

Back in July of '80, I was diagnosed as having terminal lung cancer. The doctors, there were five doctors, said I had six months, maybe a year to live. They said I had to take radiation and chemotherapy. I was supposed to have twelve treatments of radiation. I only took six. I refused the rest, and I decided that there was some way that I had to help myself.

I went to a health institute in Boston for a week and started a raw-food diet. After that I went to my twin sister's house in Connecticut. She is into health foods. Anything that was a vegetable and raw, she was juicing: carrots, parsley, celery, cabbage. I drank orange juice. She was also using grains, like lentils—sprouting them and then juicing them. I was also taking colonics. This has to do with cleansing of the colon; the colon is supposed to be a breeding ground for diseases. After two months of this, I ended up in the hospital.

The cancer started to grow and I was losing my breath. Then I couldn't breathe, which was a horrible thing, but I just felt good inside. I was ready. I remember I wanted to die; I would say, "God, I'm ready, come and take me." For two days, I lay in the hospital, not able to breathe: I knew I was dying. I don't know what happened because all of a sudden—Whammo!—my breath came back, just like that. To me, it was God's doing. He just didn't want me.

I did get a taste of death, and that's why I'm not afraid anymore. To get up every morning and face this life is harder than dying.

I used to be afraid of everything. That God was gonna punish me for doing wrong. I was afraid of being raped or attacked. There are so many fears in life. I was always afraid of running out of money.

When the cancer spread, I was in a semiconscious mind, but I felt good inside. I got a taste of death, and that's why I'm not afraid anymore. I'm glad I had the experience; now I don't fear anything.

I think there's a better life beyond here, although life is beautiful at times. I have my two sons, and I love them deeply, and, of course, there's my husband. But he's an adult. He knows how to run his own life. My children need me. I think that's the only thing that hurts me deeply about dying.

I consider myself a very lucky person in many ways. I've got a good husband. I have two wonderful kids. I've got everything most people don't have. I mean I don't have money, but to me that's not important.

My husband and I are more aware now. Aware of what's important, aware that your life can be so happy one minute, and the next minute it could end.

I'm sure that my smoking so many years caused it. I smoked for twenty-one years. I quit two years before the diagnosis. My body went through such a reaction, it was unbelievable. When I quit, I turned to junk foods, candy, chips, all kinds of greasy food, french fries, a lot of meats. Now I try and eat good. I eat a lot of vegetables and fruit.

I still smoke. I don't believe I'm gonna get better. I figure that it will get to me sooner or later. But I do believe in miracles.

I try to keep a good mind about life. When I think about my illness, I distract it, I knock it down. I never dwell on it, no! Even when I have pain, I just chalk it up and say, "Well, we all have to suffer here."

I was always a strong-willed person. I was always someone to get things done. I was always a doer. I was never one to fall down and not pick myself up, whether I was sick or not.

I always try and be happy, never sad. If I'm sad or really depressed—I rarely get depressed—I'll smoke a joint and I'm happy. I listen to music and have happy thoughts.

I've gotten down many a time, but I don't like to be down. I don't want to be a negative person. I don't even want to be near negative people. And I can control that. I have control over everything in my life, except the cigarettes. I've tried to quit again. I don't know, I just can't quit.

I think your mind rules your body. I want to say this. It might seem strange, but I'm obsessed with something. Every day I take a real hot shower. When I get into the shower, I just point the nozzle and direct the heat from the water to that area on my chest. I just sort of meditate in the shower and say, "Kill all those bad cells, kill all those bad cells." It's an obsession with me.

The heat penetrates through my body. I'm saying to them, "Go away, go away, go away." I think it a lot. I wish the bad cells away for a few minutes. It's an obsession, and I think that it has helped. I feel so much better when I get out of the shower. It might seem strange, but to me it's natural.

I recently spoke with Carole again, nearly nine years since the original diagnosis. She remains free of cancer and is physically more active than ever. Four years ago she went through a divorce that, she says, "broke my heart." Subsequently she enrolled at a community college and took classes until financial pressures made it impossible to continue. Now she awakens at five o'clock every morning to prepare for her work as a waitress. In addition to this forty-hour-a-week job, she mothers her two teenage boys and also manages the three-family home that she recently purchased from her exhusband.

Deep relaxation and focused concentration were the most salient features of Carole's self-devised visualization approach. Many alternative healers and some MDs now teach patients visualization techniques that rely on the same core features that Carole intuitively adopted. Visualization or guided imagery attempts to influence the present situation by imagining a desired scene. People use visualization as a healing technique, hoping that the process will have some impact on their immune systems. The goal (like other techniques that involve a changed state of consciousness) is to affect the body positively through the unconscious. Visualization might be an especially direct way of communicating with our unconscious because the formation of images is considered a more "primitive" way of thinking than using words. The formation of an image is said to precede any voluntary activity (for example, imagining yourself opening the book before you open it) whereas one doesn't necessarily verbalize internally (saying to yourself "I am going to open the book") before actually opening it.

Therapists, business consultants, and employment counselors are among the professionals who teach their clients visualization. Athletes and healers, however, are probably the most frequent users of visualization techniques. Bob Hooper, an NCAA swimming champion, believes that the variable that set him apart from his competitors was not innate ability or superior training. He explains what gave him the edge:

> Starting each day before the meet, I ran the following movie through my mind. I see myself coming into the Natatorium, with three thousand cheering fans sitting in the stands and the lights reflecting off of the water. I see myself going up to the starting block, and my competitors on each side. I hear the gun go off, and can see myself diving into the pool and taking the first stroke of butterfly. I can feel myself pulling through, taking another stroke, and then another. I see myself coming to the wall, turning, and pushing off into the backstroke with a small lead. The lead gets bigger with my underwater pull. Then I push off into the breast stroke. That's my best stroke and that's where I really open it up. And then I bring it home in the freestyle. I see myself winning!
>
> I run this movie through my mind thirty-five or forty times before each meet. When it finally comes time to swim, I just get in and win.

The Simontons, who pioneered the use of visualization among cancer patients, are careful not to prescribe how someone else's image should look, but they do suggest that certain symbols may work better than others. For example, they recommend picturing the cancer cells as weak and confused, while the treatment is strong and purposeful. One of their visualization exercises would be to:

> Picture your body's own white blood cells coming into the area where the cancer is, recognizing the abnormal cells, and destroying them. There is a vast army of white blood cells. They are very strong and aggressive. They are also very smart. There is no contest between them and the cancer cells, they will win the battle.
>
> Picture the cancer shrinking. See the dead cells being carried away by the white blood cells and being flushed from your body through the liver and kidneys and eliminated in the urine and stool.

Continue to see the cancer shrinking, until it is all gone.

Occasionally patients report that in the course of visualizing their disease, they can actually see their insides with vivid reality. One such account was described in *Why Me?*, a book co-written by Garrett Porter, a nine-year-old with a malignant brain tumor, and his psychologist, Patricia Norris, Ph.D. Spaceships and rockets, familiar symbols for a boy his age, were part of the imagery arsenal. After months of missile attacks on the tumor, he reported that, for the first time, he could no longer picture it. Months later, when a CAT scan was done, the doctor wanted to know if the tumor had been surgically removed, for they could find nothing in the CAT scan except a tiny piece of calcification—a "funny white spot."

Betty Preston

Betty Preston, the last subject in this book, is also the most difficult to introduce. Words cannot easily convey the feeling of unconditional acceptance she communicates. At age seventy, she is a beautiful woman, filled with love. Expressing this love has become her purpose in life.

About fifteen years ago, Betty was in the hospital to have the defective mitral valve of her heart replaced with a plastic one. During surgery, she experienced the heart-surgery patient's ultimate nightmare: The heart-lung machine was hooked up incorrectly. Air was inadvertently pumped into her blood vessels and head. According to her cardiologist, because of this mistake she wound up with very severe brain damage. The cardiologist also indicated his surprise that she regained consciousness and estimated that her positive outcome was, at best, a 1 in 100 probability.

While unconscious, Betty had a deep near-death experience. Near-death experiences were once considered fabrications, hallucinations, and even the work of the devil. But in recent years the work of Kenneth Ring, Ph.D., Raymond Moody, M.D., Ph.D., and others has left little doubt about the frequency of this phenomenon. A well-designed Gallup poll estimated that more than eight million Americans have had near-death experiences.

These people typically report that in the course of a serious illness or following an accident, they suddenly found themselves looking down at their own bodies as if they were impartial spectators. Each near-death experience is unique, but there are common features. The usual progression of events is said to be: separating from one's body, entering a tunnel, a life review, seeing the light, and being engulfed with light. (Betty related all of these events in her account, except for a separation from her body.) The general feeling is unparalleled ecstasy.

People who have had near-death experiences say they were alert, with an awareness of events that normally would seem impossible, even if they had been conscious. Michael Sabom's research of out-of-body experiences in *Recollections of Death* is of special interest to the skeptic. Sabom, a cardiologist, gathered near-death accounts from 116 people. He compared their descriptions of events in the environment (for example, what was taking place in the next room) with the reports of medical personnel and family members. He concluded that there had been an awareness that transcended ordinary sensory abilities.

Despite the far-reaching metaphysical implications of such occurrences, the focus here is anchored in everyday life. Kenneth Ring, a professor at the University of Connecticut, has methodically researched the effects of the near-death experience on the lives of individuals. In *Heading Toward Omega,* Ring said that it "not only changes an individual's life, but often completely and radically transforms it." He concluded that the near-death experience served as a catalyst for spiritual awakening. Upon their "return," most people were unafraid of death, and this change appeared to be permanent.

Betty Preston understands what it means to live a life without fear:

In 1975 I retired from the telephone company. I had to have open-heart surgery, so I took one year to prepare myself because they said I didn't have to have it right away.

I prayed each day. My husband told me that when he got up in the morning to go to work, he just let me be because I was meditating. It was so beautiful that I didn't have one worry at all about the surgery.

I had to have a new mitral valve within my heart. During the surgery, the heart pump malfunctioned. The air, which should have been dissipated, backed up, destroying part of my brain, the part containing memories.

I imagine it happened during the operation, though I can't know. Suddenly I was wide awake. I was going around and around in a tunnel. I was not afraid. Then I saw a beautiful, beautiful light coming down the tunnel toward me. I was fascinated by it, it was so beautiful. When it came to me, it went around me and then it became me. It took everything that was wrong with me away, and I felt better than I had ever felt in my life.

Then my whole life was reviewed, like it was recorded on a computer. All of my life was shown to me: the good things, the not-so-good things. There was no condemnation. I was watching it like a bystander. Maybe it's God's way of knowing the individual or a way for me to know my life.

After my life review, down the tunnel came the most beautiful, loving light. There was the warmest most wonderful love—pure love. I felt joy and at ease. Time meant nothing. One who has not experienced it cannot know its feeling. Some people say it's Jesus; I just say that light was God. The name depends on what religion people are.

Right after that, I saw two people coming toward me, and I recognized them. They were Dr. Rudolph Dyer, he had died three years before, and Holly McKilroy, my best friend, who had died eight years before. They came to me. We were delighted to see one another. It was just a marvelous gift to get back together.

At first when I came back, I cried because I thought I had lost them again. But the experience opened me up. Now I know that any time I talk of them or think of them I can feel their presence. Like right now, I can feel their arms around me, hugging me. They're saying I'm doing a good job with this. They are my guardian angels.

During the near-death experience, they gave me all knowledge, and they told me about the future. But I wouldn't have been able to handle it and so I couldn't remember it. When something happens now, I say to myself, "Oh, I remember that."

There is no doubt that the experience was different than a dream. Other near-death experiencers feel exactly the same way. People say, "Oh, it's probably a dream." But it is so different from a dream, you know that it is real.

Right after the operation, the doctor came out and told my family that if I lived, I would be a vegetable, and my son, Bob Junior, said, "I will not accept that." He said that to a big heart doctor and to some of the other doctors, who said, "Well, no, she can't be all right." Later the heart doctor said that was the best thing that he could have done because it put doubt in his mind. I've always liked my doctors, even after this happened. Dr. Rothstein was a lovely, lovely person.

Then the doctor told them that if they had anything to say to me, to say it now. My husband fainted and my other son's wife almost did, so Bob Junior came up by himself.

While I was in a coma, my other son said to me, "Ma, I love you more than anyone else in the world." It took me two years to be able to call him in California and tell him I had heard him. He said, "Mother, I am crying hard. That's exactly what I said to you, and I am so thrilled that it made a difference."

It did make a difference, because otherwise I would have stayed in that beautiful place. Not everyone has a choice, but I was far gone and I could have stayed there. I certainly wanted to, because it's so lovely and so warm and so loving.

I was in a coma for eight days. When I woke up, I knew that I was in the hospital, but I didn't know why. I had lost ten or twenty years of memory, and most of it is still gone. My friends and family all looked about ten years older. The doctors said that I could have been devastated because I couldn't walk or couldn't talk; I had to learn all over again. But I never felt devastated. I had the experience, so I knew what life is about. There was no fear.

I talk to people on the street. I say hello to almost everyone. When my husband and I were in a restaurant or someplace public, I'd nod and smile and say hello, and he'd say, "Do you have to talk to everyone?"

I'd say, "Yes. That's my job, you know."

He died a few years ago. He was a diabetic and he also drank. He lost one leg one year; the next year, he lost the other, just below the knee. It was a horrible time for me, as well as for Bob and our children. I don't know why that experience was necessary. When he decided he wanted to die, he quit eating, and he starved himself to death at the hospital.

But before that, at the hospital, he'd often talk to people who were dying, and he would say, "My wife has had a beautiful experience." He would say, "Honey, will you tell them about it."

I'd say, "All right, Bob." So I'd start talking to them, and he'd be wheeling his wheelchair away because he didn't want to hear it again. He'd wave to me, then he'd go on, and I'd talk to the people there. It is so wonderful to be able to tell people that are really hurting that there really is nothing to worry about.

I have absolutely no fear any longer. I never worry about tomorrow or anything else because I know that it's going to be all right. In fact, I had a heart attack when I was here in California last New Year's; at that time, I told the doctor if I should stop breathing, please let me go this time.

I came back to teach and be unconditional love. This was my job, but it took me a long time to be able to do it well. At first I tried to tell people what I experienced; but I would stutter, and lots of times people would turn around and walk away not to embarrass me. But I knew that's what I came back for—to be and to teach unconditional love.

Everywhere I go I try and help people. If I find someone is not interested in my story, I don't bother them. I only talk to people who are eager to hear what I have to say.

I visit at hospitals. Some people don't have anything to hold onto except their own self; and their own self isn't doing well, so they're scared. I think it makes a big difference to have faith in something— God or whatever you want to call it.

Everybody has a healing power with them. Everyone has it. All you have to do is know it and enter into it and say, "OK, I need to be healed of this. I accept, it, I expect it, and I thank you for it."

I go to high schools and I talk with college students. I tell them not to be afraid. I tell the children to try not to hurt anyone, to try and do the very best they can with their life and to help other people because that's what life is all about. It's not about making a lot of money and having a good show of what you have. I say,

"Never ever think of taking your life because God only has that right. Otherwise you might just have to do it over again."

They always seem to be very interested in what I have to say, and they line up to give me hugs before they leave. My own doctor, the regular one that I go to from the group plan, always comes and gives me big hugs whenever I see him. It sounds like I'm looking for hugs all the time, but it just happens. I know that love shines from my face, and they can't help but love me. Because I love them, it's God within me that is loving each and every one.

OBSERVATIONS

For most people in this culture, coming to terms with death takes at least a lifetime. The fear can be so great and the prospect of peace can seem so remote that many people don't begin the quest until the evidence of their finality overwhelms them. And even when death appears imminent, fears may still make it impossible to confront the meaning of one's own death.

The premise of this discussion is that dealing with death has a profound effect on psychological, spiritual, and perhaps even physical well-being. It may seem contradictory, but, except in acute medical situations, preparing for death does not conflict with the goal of staying alive. In a personal interview, Sid Baker, medical director of the Gesell Institute of Human Development, explains:

> If people are truly in jeopardy, the question comes up whether they are dying or living. In the hospital setting, there is a conflict between helping them do one versus the other. There's a point at which you stick an endotracheal tube down somebody and blow into it and bother them a lot, and there's another point at which you hold their hand and wish them well. And you can't do both at the same time. The whole scene around a resuscitation is so awful compared to the way in which people should be permitted to die.
>
> At least in the nonacute situation, I have resolved this issue for myself. I think that the agenda for dying is to clean up your life: to say things that have been unsaid, to express feelings that have been unexpressed, to finish your

emotional business with other human beings. It turns out that is a good recipe for living. In fact, it is the recipe for living. I may say to a person in jeopardy, "Look, let's face it. You're in trouble here. You've got some metastases, and this is not good news. Here I am a doctor, and I would like you to live; but if you're going to die, there are a few things I'd like to tell you about dying. You may feel that by preparing for death, you're giving up and that you are turning your back on life. But I say, no, the task is the same. If you're going to live, you have to make some changes in yourself that have to do with being more true to yourself. And if you're going to die, you have to go around and talk to some people in ways that are more true to yourself. The paths then lead to the same point."

It's amazing how many people come back and say, "You know, this cancer or this illness has been the best thing ever to happen to me."

Existential psychologists as well as various Indian gurus articulate a connection between the individual's fear of death and all other fears. Every human fear is said to be rooted in this primal fear. If one is able to confront his own mortality and free himself from fears of death, all other fears can be eliminated. Some people hold onto their fear of death, believing that they risk death by letting go. However, the fear of death keeps us from living, not from dying.

Whether ill or not, a person's every waking moment is influenced by his or her relationship with death. Many years ago, a physician who counsels both the sick and the well drew a helpful analogy. While we sat in his office, he said, "Imagine that outside the office door is some horrible monster waiting to get you. Consider how you would feel right now in this room." He paused before continuing, "Now imagine that outside this door is paradise. It's beautiful, peaceful, and loving beyond your greatest expectations. Consider how you would feel in this room right now." Though the room remained unchanged, even in this fantasy situation my feelings about it fluctuated greatly depending on how I viewed the alternatives waiting for me. The point was made: Our beliefs about death have an immediate impact on our lives.

There is good reason to struggle with this issue. If we believe that some horrible fate is always lurking in the wings, how can life really be enjoyed? But if we live as though death marked the start of some great unknown adventure, we are freed to experience the contentment that comes from living in the moment. Suddenly there is no reason to devote so much life energy to our vigilant but futile attempts to anticipate and control the future.

Intimacy and love are the potential rewards of the dying process. But fear makes us strangers to our own feelings. To "protect" ourselves, we may stay aloof from seriously ill persons and miss the purpose of these difficult human trials. This lost potential will lead to disappointment and loneliness and it may seem that only death can spare the ordeal of tenuous life. By taking the risk and sharing our pain, anger, fear, and love, we experience the comfort and meaning of human connectedness.

In order to keep death as clinical and removed as possible, we sometimes arrange for the hospitalization of the dying, though medical treatment may not be necessary or possible. Hoping that someone other than ourselves really knows how death should be dealt with, we collude with medical professionals when we pretend that they know best. In *The Mechanic and the Gardener,* Lawrence LeShan wrote:

> We no longer even believe in our ability to die alone or in the warmth of the company of our loved one. We feel that we must have around us a court of white-coated antiseptic figures to make the final transition. The individual has come to feel so helpless that he cannot even wrestle with his own death or find his own path to it.

Even though they themselves are ambivalent, seriously ill patients with physical pain sometimes find that family members, friends, and medical personnel are encouraging them to take potent pain relievers. Relieving the patient's pain may be the conscious motive of these urgings, but the unconscious motivation may be to help everyone avoid the subject of death. If patients are euphoric, semiconscious, or sleeping constantly as a result of medication, they are unlikely to talk about their impending death. Few physicians acknowledge that they prescribe narcotics for any purpose other than to relieve pain. In *Death, Dying and Euthanasia,* Richard Lamerton says that there are times when medication is employed exclusively for the purpose of quieting fears of death. It is not only the *patient's* fears that need easing. In an article published in the *Annals of Internal Medicine,* physicians were shown to be more afraid of death than their patients.

If powerful pain medication, like the narcotics, simply removed pain, there would be no issue, but each milligram of morphine, every tablet of methadone, extracts a price. Medication distorts the way an individual experiences his or her world as the state of consciousness is altered. Consequently the common dictum that, above all else, the dying patient must be kept out of pain does not adequately respect the values and wishes of every dying patient. Empowered with a choice, some individuals opt for less medication even if it means more pain. While dying a painful death, Freud said, "I prefer to think in torment than not to be able to think."

Apathy is a common side effect of narcotic medication. In fact, the results are sometimes compared to a prefrontal lobotomy. What could be more detrimental to the individual still struggling for his very existence than a drug that induces lethargy? Ideally patients would determine the case for and against various dosages of narcotic medication. The process would be ongoing, subject to patient change at any time. In this situation, as in all features of care, the patients would make as many decisions about the process as possible, including the right to decide that they want someone else to make the decisions for them. Ideally patients would make the major decisions concerning their emotional and physical needs, reserving for themselves the absolute right to decide whether or not to talk about the prospect of death.

Though making peace with death is a lifetime of work for many people, it seems that the near-death experience is so intense that it can instantaneously produce the same results. Elisabeth Kübler-Ross, a leading authority on death and dying in the United States—if there is such a thing as an authority on death—knows the power of the near-death experience. Dr. Kübler-Ross writes from her own experiences: "Anyone who has been blessed enough to see this light will never again be afraid to die. The unconditional love, the understanding and compassion in the presence of this light are beyond any human description."

For the 95 percent of us who have known neither the gift nor the intrusion of a near-death experience, however, contemplating our death remains a matter of personal volition and requires willful intent. Ultimately this struggle is worthy of our greatest effort, for this process can bring us in touch with the essence of life. When Hassidic Rabbi Buram was on his deathbed, he asked his wife why she was crying: "My whole life was only that I might learn to die."

The power of peace is realized when we come to terms with all facets of life, including death. One spiritual tale relates an imagined show-down between Attila the Hun and Buddha. Attila and his gang have entered the monastery, killing the monks and pillaging the sanctuary. The holy men are frantically scurrying about, except for Buddha, who remains serenely seated in a lotus position. With his sword raised, Attila screams at Buddha: "Don't you know who I am? I could thrust my sword through your belly without batting an eye!"

Without flinching, the Buddha responds, "Don't you know who I am? I could take your sword into my belly without batting an eye."

To try to better understand the relationship between acceptance of death and healing, I attended a meeting of near-death experiencers. (The near-death experience has proven so powerful for many people that support groups have sprung up around the country.) The twenty mem-bers who attended were in agreement that their bodies healed faster after the near-death experience. I said that I did not understand why this would be the case. A middle-aged woman who had taken up motorcycle racing after her near-death experience responded. She described how quickly she had mended after a serious motorcycle accident and specu-lated why. She now felt attuned with her body's inherent capacity to heal itself. She no longer blocked her body's natural propensity to reestablish health.

Similar to people who have had near-death experiences, most of the survivors I interviewed seemed unafraid of death. Consequently their immune systems weren't depleted by anxiety, panic, or depres-sion while they worked toward recovery. At the deepest levels, the survivors were not distressed about the possible repercussions of their condition; they wanted to be well and worked hard for their health, but they knew that even the worst physical outcome would be all right.

This discussion could not help but be overly simplistic. Death and dying, like life and living, are too complicated to say that one has them figured out, and that's that. Those who struggle with issues of death know that there may be peace one day while, the next day, nothing makes sense. A commitment to seek understanding is all one can do.

In dying, the individual must make his or her own way. Woody Allen has said, "It's not that I am afraid of dying: I just don't want to be there when it happens." There is nothing wrong in deciding that you can't be there, but the event seems especially unlikely to be cancelled if you don't show up, and you and the people you love might miss something very special.

CONCLUSION

Two summers ago, while vacationing on Cape Cod with some friends, I nearly drowned. It was my final day of vacation, and I wanted to make the most of it. As soon as we got to the beach, I put my blanket down and ran to the water.

A storm far out in the Atlantic was whipping up large waves that were rare for Cape beaches. I felt sure it was going to be a great day because the sun was hot and the waves were incredible. Body surfing had always been a favorite activity of mine. I felt a special affinity with nature when I caught a good wave and allowed myself to "go with the flow."

I ran back to the blanket to try to persuade the others to come in, too. One friend said it would take him a few minutes to prepare for the icy Atlantic, but he would join me shortly.

As I rushed to get back in the water, I failed to notice for a second time that a red flag was flying at the unmanned lifeguard station. Because of the severe conditions, all the ocean beaches on the Cape were closed for the day.

Most of the waves were breaking very far off; not being a strong swimmer, I didn't dare go far enough out to ride the best ones. But the ocean was so turbulent that riding the foam from the spent waves was still a delight.

After about half an hour, I was chilled and signaled to my friend that I was getting out of the water. On my way in, a wave caught me unaware and knocked me down. Rather than struggle against it, I decided to go with it. After a brief ride, I tried to stand up, figuring I would walk the last couple hundred yards in to shore. But there was no ground under me.

I was not alarmed, though I didn't like to be over my head in the ocean. I swam for a couple of minutes believing that there would now be solid ground when I stood up. But again there wasn't. So I swam for a couple more minutes, and, this time, when there still was no sand under my feet, I grew uneasy.

I swam longer than before, certain that this would do it. But, again, nothing but water. I couldn't understand it; the shore still seemed so far away. I was frightened. After three more episodes of swimming and checking, I felt my heart pounding. I worked to calm myself, with some success, and continued on.

After a five-minute swim without any change, I was terrified. I had to calm myself. I turned over to float on my back to relax. Whenever I had needed to relax in the past, meditation was something I could always count on. I had been doing it regularly for thirteen years, so, despite the turbulence of the ocean, taking a minute off to meditate and regain some composure seemed to make sense. But, for the first time ever, I couldn't meditate, not even for a second.

I let myself drop to see how far down the bottom was. I couldn't find it. I felt so scared.

I was exhausted. I knew I was going to drown if I didn't get help quickly. Automatically, it seemed, I raised my hands out of the water, cupped them to my mouth, and yelled as loud as I could: "Help, help, help!" Every ounce of energy that was left went into each yell.

But I was very far from shore. I could scarcely make out people on the beach. No one was coming to help. I didn't know if they could hear me or see me; they seemed to be standing and watching.

I had blurred thoughts of my young son. He needed me; I had to see him again; I couldn't die. I kept yelling, and still no one seemed to notice me. I don't know whether the cold of the water or the panic was immobilizing me, but I could hardly move. I had no energy left even to scream. I was certain that I would die. Son or no son, there was nothing I could do.

In a fleeting moment of clarity, I knew that, at most, I had fifteen seconds left before I went under. There was no one in sight. I thought of God. These were not loving or comforting thoughts—just a vague recollection that wasn't one supposed to think of God before death? I couldn't let go, even though there seemed to be no choice but to die. I was so afraid of the first breath of water. I didn't want to die. Each moment was horrific, the worst I had ever known. It could get no worse. And yet somehow each passing second was more terrifying than the last.

Suddenly from behind I heard a voice, "Take it easy." Rick Gildea, the friend I had coaxed into coming out to play, was holding me up. Within minutes, two off-duty lifeguards appeared with their surfboards. They had been walking on the beach when they heard the screams, ran back to the shelter, and retrieved their surfboards. I was told to hang on, but I couldn't and fell off a couple of times on the way in.

Finally I was brought onto the shore, where a crowd pulled me up onto the dry sand. It was strange to see all the activity and concern because the drama had passed for me. I knew I would live. I was wrapped in a blanket and someone came running down the beach with oxygen. They didn't seem to know how to administer it, and I thought, how ironic if I had survived the near drowning only to have my brains blown out with a blast of oxygen. Soon some official emergency technicians were on the scene. An ambulance came, but I thought there was little reason to go to the hospital. One of the rescue workers drove me back to our cottage.

I was out of the water, but my hell was not over. I had always had trouble asking for any kind of assistance, even little favors. Suddenly I was dealing with the fact that I had been in the middle of the Atlantic begging for help from anyone. I was ashamed. I shouldn't have gotten myself into that situation; I should have been a better swimmer; I should have known it was dangerous. Along the way, I got similar unwelcome advice from others.

I learned that I had been caught in a riptide. I was told that with a riptide you need to allow the current to pull you away from shore and then, when you are able, you swim parallel to the current, which makes it possible to break free of this deadly force. I was unforgiving of myself. I felt that intuitively I should have known to "go with the flow"—what could have been more natural?

I was unforgiving of others as well. I learned that people on shore had indeed seen me in the water and heard me screaming. I asked why no one had come out. Those who could answer said they were too frightened. Word had quickly spread on shore that I was caught in a riptide, and the area was known by locals as especially treacherous.

I was ashamed. And yet I needed still more help. My friends who were there, loving and wonderful people, had been traumatized themselves. Undoubtedly their own powerlessness had been brought home to them as they waited to see if I would drown. It may have been my imagination, but it seemed that they were finding it too difficult to spend much time with me. I wanted them to be with me constantly, but I was too ashamed to ask.

I called the woman in Boston whom I had been seeing for nearly a year. I told her what had happened, and I wanted her to drive out. I needed her to be there. She made no offer. I called back later to explain how important it was. I didn't care that she was in the middle of her own crisis. I was still screaming for help, and she was just another person on the shore too frightened to try to pull me out. I had little room for psychic fairness; the relationship was over.

I was enraged with everything and everyone. I felt most angry at those who were closest to me. A friend insensitively but caringly suggested I take swimming lessons. I wished on him an experience like mine.

If I was really loved, how could this happen to me? Calling my mother and telling her about the events felt surreal. I didn't understand how she couldn't already know what I had been through. If there really were deep connections between loved ones, why hadn't she felt a thing when I was in the water?

The fact that I had survived didn't seem to matter. My ordeal and my survival felt like random events. I had nothing to do with it. More awful, God had nothing to do with it. By chance, someone had arrived in the nick of time.

Those closest to me said that perhaps the events were not just a coincidence. They attempted to remind me that I was indeed alive and physically well. But I was filled with rage that such a thing could happen, that we live such ridiculous lives. God was not loving, not vengeful, just indifferent. There was no rhyme or reason to anything.

All was random. I didn't know if I could live in such a world. I didn't know if I wanted to.

Before the accident, I had been reading a book called *Meditation and the Art of Dying*. Ever since I had become an adult I had had, for some reason, a strong interest in death and dying. Through my years of work, I believed that I had achieved some acceptance of my own mortality. I was now more frightened than ever of dying. When I took a shower, when it rained, whenever I exerted myself and became short of breath, I felt waves of panic that death would strike at any moment. I threw out the book and just wanted all thoughts of death to go away.

I had a need to tell my story, though with each telling I felt renewed shame that I had let the accident happen. If I told the story enough, perhaps I could awaken from the nightmare. For weeks, I felt as if I were screaming for help, and still no one would come out into the water with me. Still worse, I didn't know if anyone could even hear me. There were days when I felt so alone and so afraid that I didn't know if I should thank my rescuers or curse them.

Now when I work with a person who is seriously ill, I marvel at how simple my trauma was in comparison. My hell lasted thirty minutes, an hour at most. I can't imagine how someone confronts, day after day, a critical illness. The feeling that he or she is in physical danger is not merely an illusion. There is no dream from which to awaken.

My experience in the Atlantic and the research I've done have led me to believe that we can never know in advance how we will respond to a life-threatening illness or accident. We certainly don't know how someone else *should* respond. That doesn't mean, however, that our presence isn't vitally important to the person who is ill. The sick individual needs to be listened to, cared for, and loved. Listening is not an easy task when what we want to do is to rescue the people we love from their illness and their pain. Yet, if we can do neither, the discomfort of our human limitations may seem unbearable. We may react by telling the other person what he or she should do, or by fleeing.

The people of this book have good reason to consider themselves experts at exceptional survival. And, although they adamantly believe in the efficacy of their own methods, they do not propose that their ways would necessarily be successful for anyone else. When asked how they might counsel a friend or relative who had a disease similar to their own, all declined to give specific advice. They certainly would not attempt to prescribe a treatment plan for another seriously ill patient. The action that the survivors chose to take in their own cases originated from within; they know that the most valuable help they can offer is to encourage the ill person's self-understanding. Their experience has demonstrated that each individual must discover for himself or herself what is life-giving.

There is always a reason to be hopeful about the future. The stories here do not mean to suggest what path to follow; rather they point out that peace and freedom are obtainable. The problem, pain, and challenge come in finding one's own way.

THE CONCLUSIONS OF OTHER INVESTIGATORS

The conclusions drawn by the people who tell their stories in this book are corroborated by the findings of other investigators. But the research into extraordinary recovery is very meager in light of its potential significance, and most of it concerns cancer survivors. The fact that there are more cancer studies does not mean that extraordinary recovery from cancer is more frequent than from other serious illnesses. The disparity is a consequence of scientific methodology. Over the years, the ways to classify cancer have been sufficiently refined to predict with some accuracy how the "typical" case is likely to respond. Compared to other diseases, then, it is generally easiest to determine when a cancer patient has done exceptionally well.

I believe that the characteristics associated with the extraordinary cancer patient are similar to the characteristics of all extraordinary patients. If recovered cancer patients are somehow different, it may be most noticeable in their ability to develop characteristics counter to those of the "cancer personality." For example, if repressed emotion is more common to people who develop cancer, then learning to express their feelings may be especially characteristic of extraordinary cancer survivors.

Japanese doctors from the school of medicine at Kyushu University reported five cases of cancer that regressed without any apparent medical explanation. In ways similar to the stories in this book, the patients assumed responsibility for their illness and the quality of their lives. All five people developed a dramatically different outlook on life as they seemed to let go of worldly attachments and got closer to their "true nature." This team of four researchers concluded that "mere coincidence" did not account for the recovery of these people.

Dr. Kenneth Pelletier also found that extraordinary survivors positively changed their innermost sense of themselves. Meditation, prayer, or other revelatory experience seemed to precipitate these changes. In general, they took better care of their bodies, and, more specifically, they all made significant dietary changes.

Judith Glassman, a medical journalist, interviewed cancer patients in depth. She states that those who were determined to be the exception were also the ones most likely to accomplish exceptional recoveries. Patients who recovered actively participated in their treatment decisions and used their physicians as consultants. Survivors "were able to battle their disease and, if necessary, their doctors, friends, and family. . . . It is not the placid, quiet, agreeable 'good' patient who recovers but the crabby, ornery, cantankerous one."

These patients did not deny their feelings. As one of Glassman's interviewees said:

> The emotions are always right. . . . I feel that was one of the essentials in my healing: I felt exactly what I felt. When I was first diagnosed everybody kept saying to me, "You've got to have a good attitude," and I kept saying to myself, "How am I going to get it?" If you don't own your emotions, you're not going to make it. Be negative if that's how you feel. If you don't acknowledge what is, you can't change.

Charles Weinstock, M.D., researched twelve different cases of "spontaneous regression." All the patients that he studied shared one common emotion—hope. At the University of Minnesota Medical School, Dr. B. J. Kennedy and his associates studied twenty-two patients who had been cured of advanced cancer. From the beginning of their illnesses, patients reported confidence that they could recover and generally believed in their doctors and treatment. The survivors had a better self-image and felt more appreciative of life and other people than did the individuals in three control groups.

Similarly, the Simontons found that patients who become actively involved in their treatment, who trust their ability to influence the disease, and who develop a better self-image are most likely to get well.

In a study just completed, medical faculty members from Erasmus University in the Netherlands researched the "spontaneous regression" of six cancer patients. By interviewing the subjects' family members, where possible, Drs. Daan van Baalen and Marco de Vries sought to establish that the subjects' changes preceded their cures and thus were not a result of their unusual recoveries. The researchers found that extraordinary survivors, unlike those with advanced progressive cancer, made specific changes in their daily routines, especially dietary changes. Internally they began to feel less helpless and more autonomous, and, because of these positive changes, they also interacted less passively with medical personnel, spouses, and other family members. They developed more caring relationships than previously. Like the people in *Making Miracles,* these survivors made radical existential shifts.

The results of these studies are all strikingly similar: What differences there are basically reflect the researcher's particular emphasis. Bernie Siegel's message is entirely consistent with these findings. He, however, uses a language that more fully embraces the spiritual dimensions of healing: "Acceptance, faith, forgiveness, peace and love are the characteristics which always appear in those who achieve unexpected healing of serious illness. . . . If one loves enough, anything can be accomplished."

People who have survived "terminal" illness and people who have survived lethal environments share some basic qualities. For example, the few who lived through the horrors of the Nazi concentration camps remained hopeful despite the hopelessness of the situation. In *None of Us Will Return,* Charlotte Delbo offers a graphic depiction of the differences in attitudes between the narrator and another prisoner:

> "There's no hope for us."
> And her hand makes a gesture and the gesture evokes rising smoke.
> "We must fight with all our strength."

"Why?... Why fight since all of us have to..." The hand completes the gesture. Rising smoke.

"No. We must fight."

"How can we hope to get out of here? How could anyone ever get out of here? It would be better to throw ourselves on the barbed wire right now."

What is there to say to her? She is small, sickly. And I am unable to persuade myself. All arguments are senseless. I am at odds with my reason. One is at odds with all reason.

Counter to rational logic, those who gave the most of themselves fared the best in the death camps. Giving to others actually aided survival. In *The Survivor,* Terence Des Pres quotes a Treblinka survivor: "In our group we shared everything; and the moment one of the group ate something without sharing it, we knew it was the beginning of the end for him." Those who continued to live consistently served others. According to Stephen Levine, they were the "doctors, the nuns, the priests, the rabbis, the mothering and fathering care-givers. They survived because they had a reason to live: love itself, healing itself. They knew that love is the only gift worth giving. That our care for others is our care for ourselves, a deep honoring of the being we all share." Love brought meaning to the concentration camp survivors and to the survivors of serious illness.

THE NEED TO CHANGE

When one is facing danger, the natural human tendency is to hold onto old ways more tightly than ever, even though these old ways may actually contribute to the problem. To find peace, however, it is often necessary to let go and discover a new way of experiencing reality. Survivors consistently tell us that they underwent an existential shift in thinking, a fundamental change in the way they viewed their existence. They incorporated death and dying as a natural and necessary part of life. If death ceases to be the enemy, a tragedy, or a failure, one soon recognizes that everything is happening just the way it should. That does not mean we stop striving, only that we strive without attachment to the outcome. Zen Master Szuki Roshi put it this way, "Everything is perfect, but there is always room for improvement."

When individuals are fighting for their very lives, the idea that some can do more than just attempt to get through the next moment seems incredible. Yet extraordinary survivors have used their afflictions as a signal to change in the most profound ways possible. Indeed, many others who are ill also accomplish a psychological and spiritual healing without ever realizing a physical cure.

Before the onset of disease, many of the survivors described their lives as empty, devoid of any real meaning. Some were lost in their deep psychic pain, and a few saw the disease as a physical manifestation of the pain. Often, the first step toward recovery was finding a purpose in life. The source of meaning was varied: The relationships that Phina Dacri and Leo Perras had with God proved sustaining; music gave Joe Godinski a reason to live, while survival itself became a powerful source of meaning for Kurt Metzler.

For the vast majority of extraordinary survivors I have met, a loving relationship fuels their fight to stay alive. In many instances, survivors have a partner with whom they share an intense commitment. The wife of a survivor, a seventy-two-year-old woman, actually participated in some forms of her husband's "treatment." After his "terminal" prognosis, the couple searched desperately for an elixir. This woman described their experiment with an unknown tea:

> We heard about this tea that was supposed to cure cancer.
> But how did we know if it was poison or not? The FDA was
> trying to catch the guy who was distributing it. So I said to
> Carl, "If you're going to drink it, then I'm going to drink it.
> If you're going to be poisoned, I'm going to be poisoned." So
> we ordered enough tea for each of us to drink for a few
> weeks.

The people of *Making Miracles* seized the illness as an opportunity to make dramatic changes in their personal relationships. They expressed their emotions—especially angry and loving feelings—more readily than they had before, which enabled them to form more intimate relationships. Thus they gave more but also expected more than in the past. In some instances, they found it necessary to dissolve relationships that held little promise of fulfillment.

Physicians played a significant role in the healing process. Recovery, however, was not attributed to the technical or mechanical expertise of doctors. Patient after patient asserts that it was the loving care that helped to heal them. The relationships that a few had with their doctors actually became a reason to stay alive. For example, when Lindsey Reynolds felt most despondent, she said it was her psychiatrist's love that kept her from taking her life.

Survivors followed their hearts' passions after they became ill. Living this way was so satisfying that they didn't regress to old patterns once they recovered. Joe Godinski stopped selling encyclopedias and became a jazz musician; Raymond Berté moved out of the city onto a farm; Walter Purington left a job he had disliked for thirty-five years. Facing a tenuous future, they chose to live in the here and now. As Phina Dacri said, "My life is beautiful now. I used to wake up and say, 'Ho, hum, another day.' Now I wake up and say, 'Thank you, God.'" Their lives—all life—took on a preciousness never known before.

They discarded the stress of trying to live up to some external standard. They felt less obliged to please others or act as they thought they were supposed to. When an elderly Quaker was asked if his illness might have offered new freedom, he responded, "That's for sure. I had tried to be a spiritually centered person all my life. But I've tried it so tensely and so introspectively that there probably have been as many problems as good arising from it." In general, since the prognosis, these people have done a remarkable job of letting go of previously learned behaviors and attitudes that stifled their unique individual expression.

Like concentration camp survivors, their confidence defied rational logic. The optimism of many was unequivocal, even though their bleak prognoses carried the full authority of medical science. Walter Purington declared, "I never thought I wasn't going to get better," while Joe Godinski could say, "That's ridiculous. I'm not going to have that," even though statistics suggested it would take a miracle to get better once his cancer had spread to his brain and eye. Some saw the illness as a challenge that they knew they would conquer. Norman Cousins explained: "The term 'irreversible' really set off a fire inside me. I can still feel the terrific surge. There's a certain amount of joy that comes from knowing that you're going to win no matter what may be involved."

Of course, each experienced times of questioning, wondering if recovery or continued life was really possible. Individuals were most vulnerable shortly after the diagnosis, and a recurrence of the disease triggered doubts about the path they had chosen. An occasional bout of depression was not uncommon, but generally they felt optimistic about their ability to influence their disease.

Hope was not simply something that the people in these stories were blessed with; they constructed external environments that would support the frame of mind they were attempting to create. For example, Barbara Dawson visited countless doctors until she found one who would offer at least a shred of hope; Leo Perras kept people around him who believed that anything was possible, while Carole Matthews stayed away from people who were not positive; Walter Purington made an emotional journey far from his familiar Yankee setting to engage a Tibetan doctor who said cure was possible.

THE INDIVIDUALITY OF HEALING

The preceding discussion may offer some interesting and provocative generalizations about the experience of survivors. But there is a danger: These generalizations can minimize and even distort the very distinct nature of each person's healing process. As a matter of fact, all those interviewed adopted certain behaviors and beliefs that were different from the others as they listened to their unconscious, tuned into their bodies, and determined what course of action to follow.

My interview with Lloyd Schmidt, a retired asbestos worker, demonstrates the idiosyncrasy of healing. Soon after contracting inoperable lung cancer with tracheal involvement, Lloyd developed brain metastasis (median survival is only four months). I interviewed him approximately five years after the diagnosis, and his oncologist wrote: "He was treated with a palliative (noncurative) dose of radiation, and in a most unusual fashion, he has remained well without evidence of disease since then. His chances of surviving until now were approximately 1 in 1,000." Although Lloyd died last year at the age of sixty-three, about eight years after his cancer was identified, his longevity would be considered outstanding by any measure.

Lloyd viewed his cancer as tiny bugs attempting to devour him. His course of action was consistent with this belief system:

> They told me I had about seven months to live, but I
> decided for myself that they were all wrong. . . . I was deter-

mined to eat a lot and let the cancer chew on something besides me. I ordered three orders of everything while I was in the hospital getting these twenty-four cobalt treatments. I ate a lot of fruits and vegetables, custard and jello. They'd have grapefruit for breakfast. I put down three bowls of grapefruit, and they'd have custard and ice cream for dinner, and I'd put down five custards. . . . And at night I'd order extra so I'd have something before I went to sleep. I had the top of the radiator all lined up with milk. They couldn't believe how much I was eating. The dietician from the hospital, she didn't believe that anyone could consume that much. She came up to watch me eat a couple of meals. I just said, "I'm gonna let that cancer eat a lot of fat before it eats me."

During treatment that causes other patients to lose their appetites and become emaciated and malnourished, this man gained fifty-five pounds and seemed to thrive.

The differences in thought and action are plentiful enough to conclude that there are very few, if any, universal characteristics of all extraordinary patients. For example, as a group they were adamant about the need to direct and control their own treatment. But Phina Dacri said that she simply put all her faith in her doctors and never even asked them any questions. Similarly, there was a consensus that diet played a significant role in the exceptional results. Joe's breakfast during the interview, however—coffee, white toast and bacon and eggs, topped off with a cigarette—supported his assertion that his eating habits were not a factor in his healing.

THE WILL TO LIVE AND LOVE

It is generally agreed by physicians and lay people alike that the patient's will to live can influence any serious illness. Yet medical scientists do not research its effects, doctors do not study it in medical school, and neither doctor nor patient consciously enlist this immense reservoir of healing potential to help fight devastating illness.

How do we explain this paradox?

Medical personnel, like the rest of us, usually underestimate the capacity of humans to change and grow. One's very life source, the will to live, is often considered to be out of the individual's control. There is no reason, then, for the patient or physician to try to invoke the power of the will to live, for it's either part of a person's inherent makeup or it isn't. Those who have recovered from life-threatening illness or catastrophic accident know otherwise.

"I didn't really care about living until they told me I was going to die," a middle-aged survivor confided, but the sentiment reflects the feelings of many extraordinary patients. The people of this book tell us that the desire to live evolved over time. They made internal and external changes that transformed their lives. They learned to forgive themselves and accept who they were, which made it possible for them to love themselves and to love others. Living in love, there was no ambivalence about being alive. Continued life was worth their best effort. They had reason to devote themselves to the healing process, and the more they worked at it, the stronger their desire grew to stay alive.

The implications here are significant for everyone—not just the seriously ill. The people in this book gained insight into far more than just what would sustain their lives. They discovered how to live. Their secrets were not esoteric formulas for physical healing. They learned how to appreciate each moment of their existence. Clearly they had a powerful motivation to change. But their message is that we do not need to wait until catastrophe strikes to come in touch with our essence, to find meaning in our lives. We all have the power to affect our existence in the most profound ways imaginable.

These people opened themselves to love. They witnessed their own inner beauty and knew that they were worthy of being loved. They felt loved by God, loved by people special to them, and learned to love themselves—and so were attuned with the ultimate truth. In the midst of horrendous struggles that they could have interpreted as meaningless blows of fate, they experienced the perfection of the universe.

Moments of pure consciousness, of awareness, of love, lead to psychological and spiritual healing and allow for physical healing. Love transcends death. Parents who would step in harm's way to save their child's life or anyone who has even imagined sacrificing his life for another knows that love is stronger than our supposed most basic human instinct for self-preservation. Nothing is more powerful.

As Pierre Teilhard de Chardin said, the power of love may be limitless: "Someday, after we have mastered the winds, the waves, the tides and gravity, we shall harness for God the energies of love. Then for the second time in the history of the world, man will have discovered fire."

Love transcends death, which doesn't mean that love will restore our bodies, but it can. Yet if love doesn't sustain the body and one dies in love, the individual has still realized the highest purpose of life.

Sample Questionnaire Completed by Physicians

1. When the patient's most serious diagnosis was confirmed, the consensus of medical opinion would probably suggest that the likelihood of survival for

(a) longer than twelve months was approximately?:

(please √ along the continuum)

(1 in 1,000) very rare	(1 in 100) rare	(5 in 100) very unlikely	(10 in 100) unlikely	(25 in 100) not expected but not very unusual	(50 in 100) about even	(>50 in 100) better than even

(b) longer than three years was approximately?:

(1 in 1,000) very rare	(1 in 100) rare	(5 in 100) very unlikely	(10 in 100) unlikely	(25 in 100) not expected but not very unusual	(50 in 100) about even	(>50 in 100) better than even

(c) longer than five years was approximately?:

(1 in 1,000) very rare	(1 in 100) rare	(5 in 100) very unlikely	(10 in 100) unlikely	(25 in 100) not expected but not very unusual	(50 in 100) about even	(>50 in 100) better than even

2. If your own estimation about the probability of survival was significantly different from the consensus, please summarize your prognosis and rationale.

3. Please describe, in general terms, the patient's course of illness, treatment, and complications, if any.

4. Optional question: Do you have any impression why this person did better than anticipated?

Physicians Responses to Questionnaires

The purpose of the following information is to document that at least one medical authority considered each subject's course of illness extraordinary. In most cases, this verification comes from a questionnaire completed by the subject's physician. When appropriate, physicians were asked to cite a probability for survival. There is a range of statistical improbability among the subjects who tell their stories in this book. In the least unusual case (from a statistical perspective), the physician believed the likelihood of survival was 25 percent, while, in some other cases, the physicians labeled the recoveries "miraculous." There is nothing absolute about the estimates. Another physician might have assigned a higher or lower probability.

The medical situation (that is, the type of disease, the extent of disease, the patient's health at the time of diagnosis, the patient's age, and other factors) was different for each subject. Hence the questionnaires were similar, but, in order to elicit the most relevant information, they were not necessarily identical. In those instances in which a physician did not specifically assign a probability, other medical information has been included to indicate the unusual nature of the course of illness.

RAYMOND BERTÉ

1. Estimating the probability of survival:

The physician indicated that when the most serious diagnosis was confirmed, the likelihood of survival for longer than five years was approximately 25 in 100. [**Author's note:** Raymond has survived for more than eleven years since this diagnosis.]

2. The physician's response when asked if this probability was significantly different from medical consensus:

"A prognosis was difficult to establish because of the problem of classification of the lymphoma. Given the extent of disease at diagnosis, including marrow and peripheral blood changes, I expected a shorter survival."

3. The physician's description of the patient's illness and treatment:

"Diagnosis was made 9/22/77 by lymph node and bone marrow biopsy.

"There was a difference of opinion regarding the exact histology among the pathologists. Some reported lymphoma, diffuse, poorly differentiated; others lymphoma, diffuse, moderately well differentiated. The presentation was similar to those with nodular lymphomas and the clinical course was most consistent with the lymphoma of moderately well-differentiated type (median survival 5–7 years). The median of the diffuse poorly differentiated type is 1–2 years."

4. Physician's response when asked for any impression of why the patient did better than anticipated:

"The pathologist reporting the most favorable type of histology was correct. Additional node biopsy might have detected a more benign histology—perhaps of the nodular type with the most favorable prognosis. Predicting survival in patients with lymphoma can be most difficult and inaccurate given the wide range of histologic types and variation in aggressiveness of disease." [Note: The oncologist completed this questionnaire approximately five years after Berte's diagnosis.]

Author's Comment: The reporting oncologist indicated that there were differences of opinion regarding the exact diagnosis. Although he now believes that the less lethal (that is, longer median survival) diagnosis was correct, he still indicated that Raymond had only a 25 percent chance of surviving for five years. It is interesting to note that despite his present assumption that the less lethal diagnosis was accurate, medical personnel who were involved at the time of the diagnosis probably assumed that the more lethal diagnosis was accurate since Raymond was told that he had only six to eighteen months to live.

PHINA DACRI

1. Estimating the probability of survival:

The physician indicated that when the most serious diagnosis was confirmed, the likelihood of survival for longer than three years was approximately 5 in 100. [**Author's note:** Phina has survived for more than eleven years since this diagnosis. She remains cancer free.]

2. The physician's response when asked if this probability was significantly different from medical consensus:

"Not different. Good patient attitude and desire for survival despite poor overall odds."

3. The physician's description of the patient's illness and treatment:

"Initial diagnosis—8/78 inoperable adeno lung cancer.
"Initial symptoms—7/78 chest pain (diagnosis was myocardial infarction, but incorrect diagnosis).
"Radiation—with curative intent, 6000 rads from 9/5/78–10/31/78.
"Minimal symptoms of radiation, cough without production and no complications.
"Also had bouts of cervical spine arthritis and gallbladder problems."

4. Physician's response when asked for any impression of why the patient did better than anticipated:

"Patient accepted her diagnosis—she was told she was incurable. The severity of the diagnosis was never shielded from her but was put in perspective. She was encouraged to look to the future, not the past. She carried on, fostered a positive attitude through her treatment and is now well.''

NORMAN COUSINS

Statements from physicians in *The Healing Heart* indicate the initial severity of Norman Cousins's condition and his extraordinary course of recovery.

William Hitzig, M.D., Cousins's longtime family physician, said that in December 1980, he received a call from Dr. Kenneth Shine stating that Cousins had been brought by ambulance to the UCLA hospital in "desperate" condition: "The enzyme count, measuring the amount of heart-muscle destruction, was very high. So was the MB fraction, another important indicator. There was confirmation of fluid in his lungs. He was coughing up blood. I could understand why I had been told his condition was 'touch and go.'''

A week later, Dr. Hitzig said that Cousins's room, now filled with books, papers, and a typewriter, resembled an editorial office more than a hospital room. He commented, "I wondered how anyone who had suffered the kind of heart attack he experienced could be so strong and confident in manner. And again I thought back on my own long experience as a cardiologist and internist; I could find no parallel.''

Hitzig is aware that recoveries such as Cousins's can lead doctors to doubt the accuracy of the original diagnosis:

> I have no doubt that some of my colleagues will question whether the myocardial infarction and congestive heart failure really took place, in view of his excellent present condition....I confess that I myself find it difficult to believe that anyone who has been hit by a myocardial infarction and congestive heart failure could have come through the experience as he has done. [Written approximately two years after his heart attack.]

Dr. William Shine from the UCLA hospital corroborated the seriousness of his disease:

> The electrocardiographic and enzyme changes all indicated
> a very significant heart attack. Before he left the hospital, we
> did an exercise test on him, and that made us very concerned,
> because instead of having an increase in blood pressure, which
> one would expect from exercise, he had had a decrease. That
> was a finding of considerable seriousness, and I so informed
> him.

According to David Cannom, M.D.: "The fact of arterial blockage was incontestable. The prevailing view among cardiologists is that reversibility is very rare." But after six months of Cousins's self-devised program, he retook the treadmill test. Dr. Cannom explained that there was "a complete reversal from the treadmill experience at UCLA half a year earlier. The ominous changes on the cardiograph were now absent. There was no drop in blood pressure. An indisputable change had occurred after half a year of the rehabilitation program."

JOE GODINSKI

1. Estimating the probability of survival:

The physician indicated that when the most serious diagnosis was confirmed, the likelihood of survival for longer than twelve months was approximately 1 in 1,000. [**Author's note:** Joe has survived for more than fourteen years since this original diagnosis; he remains free of cancer.]

2. The physician's response when asked if this probability was significantly different from medical consensus:

"I believe that people are not statistics. Joe's survival did not surprise me, because "in the face of uncertainty, there is nothing wrong with hope.""

3. The physician's description of the patient's illness and treatment:

"About eight years ago, Joe was diagnosed with lung cancer (oat cell). [The physician completed the questionnaire six years ago.] He had one lobe of his left lung removed, received radiation, refused chemo.

"Then about one year later he developed a brain metastasis, treated with radiation. Then he developed a tumor behind his right eye. Treated with radiation.

"He went to the Simontons', did a lot of work on himself and healed completely. His healing is, by any standard, a miracle."

4. Physician's response when asked for any impression of why the patient did better than anticipated:

"I believe that Joe went through a psychospiritual transformation that resulted in his healing. Let's say that his 'will to live' became very strong and certain psychoneuroimmunological pathways enhanced his host resistance to the degree that he was able to eliminate cancer from his body."

LINDSEY REYNOLDS

Assessing the unusualness of a particular recovery from severe mental illness is difficult and imprecise. In a case such as Lindsey's, there was no pathology to examine under a microscope, analyze, and compare with other similarly diseased specimens. To diagnose, mental health professionals rely on observable behavior and make inferences about the patient's internal state based in part upon the clinician's intuitive feelings. In light of these considerations and the length of time elapsed since her illness (more than twenty-five years since onset), the completion of a statistically based questionnaire would yield little meaningful data. As noted in the introduction to Lindsey's story, mental health professionals did indicate the unusual nature of her recovery, though the data available for their consideration was necessarily circumscribed by the passage of time.

It was possible to substantiate the major events that Lindsey described in her narrative by examining her medical records and speaking with her psychiatrist. The following excerpts were taken directly from her Riverview Hospital (a pseudonym) medical records.

Each note was dated and signed by a physician. The intent is not to present a chronology of her illness (hence many of her admission and discharge notes are not included) but to offer selected portions of the medical record.

3/20/61——First Riverview psychiatric hospital admission of this 20-year-old college student who presents a long history (4–6 years) of episodic depression and erratic behavior.... Today she admitted to extreme depression and anxiety, last night brooding on her father's death five years ago, visiting his grave. She lacerated her wrists and thighs with bottle fragments... definite suicide risk.

5/2/62——This is the second psychiatric admission of this 20-year-old female who entered after lacerating left wrist.... Following a date on which she drank moderatedly, became depressed and felt like killing herself....
MENTAL STATUS EXAM
Impression: The gradual onset, the extensive symptomatology and its re-exacerbation (although delusions and hallucinations are not elicited) are consistent with acute, undifferentiated schizophrenia.
Diagnosis: Schizophrenic reaction, acute undifferentiated type.
Prognosis: Poor

5/16/62——Cut wrists with a razor blade that she had hidden under floor tiles.

5/20/62——Patient and her room thoroughly scrutinized, bathroom locked, patient placed on a mat on the floor. She set the cuff of her pajamas on fire.

5/25/62——The four shock treatments which patient has received to date have produced no appreciable change in affective or behavioral spheres; indeed, today, for the second time in 48 hours, the patient has indulged her compulsive penchant for self-laceration. She will be shocked on three successive days.

6/9/62——Following phone call to mother, patient broke light bulb and cut her wrist. She states that she wants to die.

6/11/62——It has been determined that electric shock can be of little or no value to patient and that in view of her continued depression, impulsive self-mutilation and persistent suicidal ruminations, long term inpatient care is the only practical approach.

8/14/63——Patient admitted today [from the emergency room] following an injury to her forehead occasioned by a fall in her apartment last night. The fall occurred in bathroom while the patient was holding a glass (probably responsible for laceration). . . . The laceration was sutured.

9/8/63——22-year-old female with a long psychiatric history (8 admissions in past 3 years) admitted to emergency in coma following ingestion of massive amounts of barbituate in deliberate suicide attempt.

10/2/63——Patient discharged today to mother, who over my protests transferred patient to Adolescent Treatment Center.

3/21/65——This patient is a chronic schizophrenic who was admitted to emergency room following an overdosage of Tuinal and aspirin. There have been many such incidents.

4/13/66——SURGICAL CONSULT
25-year-old female who while on pass this afternoon "swallowed glass," apparently a broken jelly glass. At present, complains of slight sore throat and floating abdominal pains. . . . X-ray reveals the possibility of foreign body in region of stomach. Will continue conservative regime of watchful waiting.

10/19/66——DISCHARGE SUMMARY
25-year-old white female with history of multiple hospitalizations and diagnosis of undifferentiated schizophrenia was readmitted because of loss of impulse control and suicidal impulses—patient was slow to improve, but then showed gradual response in past few days. She has handled passes and overnite well, feels anxious, but suicidal impulses are gone. She can be discharged since hospital tends to promote regressive behavior and feelings.

WALTER PURINGTON

Physician #1

1. Estimating the probability of survival.

The physician indicated that when the most serious diagnosis was confirmed, the likelihood of survival for longer than twelve months was approximately 1 in 1,000. [**Author's note:** Walter has survived for more than eight years since this diagnosis. He remains cancer free.]

2. The physician's response when asked if this probability was significantly different from medical consensus:

"I was not caring for patient at time of diagnosis, but there was consensus that his prognosis was poor." [**Author's note:** This physician began treating Walter after the diagnosis.]

3. The physician's description of the patient's illness and treatment:

"Initial admission was in 8/81 for arm and spinal pain. During that admission spinal fluid showed undifferentiated neoplastic cells in great proliferation. Gallium scan showed increased uptake in sphenoid sinus. Was given radiation treatments in 9/81 to skull and mid thoracic spine. Following completion of X-ray therapy returned home with poor prognosis.

"Was referred to hospice for terminal care and acupuncturist for Rx of pain."

4. Physician's response when asked for any impression of why the patient did better than anticipated:

"Following involvement with acupuncture, he seemed to show steady improvement when he was finally discharged from the hospice program."

Physician #2

1. Estimating the probability of survival:

The physician indicated that when the most serious diagnosis was confirmed, the likelihood of survival for longer than three years was approximately 1 in 1,000.

2. The physician's response when asked if this probability was significantly different from medical consensus:

"I concurred."

3. The physician's description of the patient's illness and treatment:

"Mr. Purington presented with abnormalities of neurological function (cranial nerve paresis) secondary to what was believed to be cancer involving the meningeal space.

"He was treated once with chemotherapy and then with radiation to the brain and spinal cord.

"He gradually improved despite the absence of further therapy. No further evidence of cancer has yet appeared." [This questionnaire was completed approximately two years after the original diagnosis.]

4. Physician's response when asked for any impression of why the patient did better than anticipated:

"The pathology of his spinal fluid was reviewed both locally and by a national expert—both of whom concurred on the diagnosis of cancer. My present assumption is that though the cells appear cancerous under the microscope, they instead represent an atypical response to some bizarre infectious process."

Author's Comment: Despite this assumption, the reporting oncologist still labelled Walter's recovery a 1 in 1,000 possibility. A consulting physician who reviewed this questionnaire said that it appears that the oncologist's questions about whether the disease was cancer or some "bizarre" infection arose only after Walter recovered. The consultant explained, "Otherwise, one has to wonder: Why didn't they attempt to treat the infectious process, especially in light of the fact that the cancer diagnosis was considered hopeless?"

KURT METZLER

Physician #1

1. Estimating the probability of survival:

The physician indicated that when the cystic fibrosis diagnosis was confirmed, the likelihood of survival until age thirty was approximately 1 in 1,000. [**Author's note:** Kurt is thirty-one years old.]

2. The physician's description of the patient's illness and treatment:

"Kurt has had a slow but progressive loss of lung function over the years, punctuated by bouts of bronchitis at times requiring intravenous antibiotic therapy and/or hospitalization. Kurt has remained very active over the years, trying to keep fit with regular exercise. He is still not significantly disabled by his illness."

3. Physician's response when asked for any impression of why the patient did better than anticipated:

"Good luck?
"Good physical conditioning?"

Physician #2

1. Estimating the probability of survival:

The physician indicated that when the cystic fibrosis diagnosis was confirmed, the likelihood of survival until age thirty was approximately 1 in 100.

2. The physician's description of the patient's illness and treatment:

"Diagnosed in infancy due to G.I. disease and failure to thrive. Over the last 15 years, progressive chronic lung disease with bronchiectasis, hemoptysis and pneumothorax have been major problems. Daily therapy is aimed at maintaining nutrition and pulmonary drainage. Exacerbations of lung disease are treated with antibiotics and may require hospitalization. His disease is slowly progressive and is expected to be life shortening—limited by progressing lung damage.''

3. Physician's response when asked for any impression of why the patient did better than anticipated:

''Supportive family, good attitude toward maintaining his health and exercise have undoubtedly contributed; however, there is a wide spectrum of disease severity among individuals as well.'' [**Author's note:** Kurt's disease is considered severe.]

LEO PERRAS

The conversation with Leo Perras's former physician (see page 174) indicates that Leo's recovery was considered extraordinary. Other sources provide corroborating information concerning the doctor's medical opinion about Leo's case:

An article in the February 1979 issue of *The Hampden Hippocrat*, a publication of the Hampden District Medical Society, discussed Leo's unusual recovery. After briefly describing the events that preceded his first steps after twenty years in a wheelchair, the article reported:

> He has been walking ever since and according to his physician, his leg muscles have essentially tripled in size. However, perhaps the most amazing thing is the complete disappearance of the pain of his back, neck and arms for which he had been taking Percodan, Seconal and occasional injections of Demerol. His problem started about 20 years ago with a low back problem for which he had two operative procedures. Following one of the procedures, he became paralyzed. Rather intractable pain of his back, arms and neck has been a major problem the past few years. A local neuro-surgeon implanted a dorsal column stimulator, but this did not ease his pain. He states that now he takes no Percodan and only occasional aspirin.

On August 29, 1978, *The Hampshire Gazette,* a regional newspaper, quoted his doctor as saying, "It is truly a miracle. . . . Neurologically, nothing has changed." The account goes on to say:

> He [the physician] recalled he was "stunned" when he saw Perras walk up to his door. . . .
>
> Although Perras is not about to run sprints with leg muscles that are atrophied from a score of sedentary years, he was walking about on his own today, moving slowly like a child taking the first steps.
>
> "His legs now are about the size of your wrists," the doctor told a reporter.

On May 23, 1979, a retrospective article in *The Hampshire Gazette* included the following excerpts:

> Perras's private doctor for 10 years said he last examined the man two months ago and discovered a 70 percent return of muscle.
>
> "Before, it was zero," he said.
>
> The doctor, also a Catholic, termed the recovery "a miracle. Neurologically, nothing has changed. It is difficult to understand."

In February 1979, *Yankee* magazine ran a brief story of Leo's recovery. According to their account:

> His family physician . . . confirmed that Perras has neither reflexes nor sensations in his legs due to a surgical procedure which had been performed earlier to relieve pain in his back. Of Perras's newfound ability to stand and walk, [his doctor] said, "Neurologically it's impossible. He's walking on legs which are so emaciated from years in a wheelchair that, anatomically, they shouldn't support him."

Later the *Yankee* magazine article stated that his physician "also remarked on the unusual recovery of Perras's atrophied leg muscles, some of which have quadrupled in size in the first three months following his first encounter with Father DiOrio."

BARBARA DAWSON

Physician #1

1. Estimating the probability of survival:

The physician indicated that when the most serious diagnosis was confirmed, the likelihood of survival for as long as she had already survived [i.e. six and a half years since the diagnosis] was approximately 1 in 1,000. [**Author's note:** Barbara Dawson's situation was considered unresolved at the time of publication.]

2. The physician's description of the patient's illness and treatment:

"Clinical diagnosis about 1980—she felt a mass.
"Pathologic diagnosis 10/8/82
"Bilateral oophorectomy 11/15/82—disease stable after that when I last saw her on 3/1/83."

3. Physician's response when asked for any impression of why the patient did better than anticipated:

"She had an indolent type of breast cancer which remained localized to breast and regional nodes for 2 years before biopsy—perhaps much longer. She apparently had a slow but good regression after hormone manipulation and these remissions are frequently good long ones.

"I wish all patients with breast cancer responded the same way."

Physician #2

1. Estimating the probability of survival:

The physician indicated that when the most serious diagnosis was confirmed, the likelihood of survival for as long as she had already survived [six and a half years since the diagnosis] was approximately 1 in 3.

2. The physician's description of the patient's illness and treatment:

"Young woman with slowly growing breast cancer, probably estrogen receptor positive, who has responded to oophorectomy.

"Her type of case is most likely to occur in a more elderly woman, who will respond to multiple hormone therapies."

3. Physician's response when asked for any impression of why the patient did better than anticipated:

"Biology of her disease."

CAROLE MATTHEWS

1. Estimating the probability of survival:

The physician indicated that when the most serious diagnosis was confirmed, the likelihood of survival for longer than three years was approximately 1 in 100. [**Author's note:** Carole has survived for more than nine years since this diagnosis. She remains disease free.]

2. The physician's response when asked if this probability was significantly different from medical consensus:

"Her actual performance in a situation of incompletely treated cancer was better than expected."

3. The physician's description of the patient's illness and treatment:

"35-year-old female, diagnosis of undifferentiated lung cancer (poor prognostic cell type) in March 1980, inoperable because of mediastinal nodal involvement.

"She completed 25 percent of the planned course of radiation to 1500 rads from 3/13 to 3/20/80. She refused further radiation, began 'diet therapy,' and refused attempts at counseling or advice. She returned in 10/80 with recurrence of her cancer and was again treated to 2100 rads from 10/17 to 10/27/80. She refused additional treatment.

"She returned with a second recurrence and allowed treatment from 4/27/81 to 5/8/81.... She has given up diet or other quackery as therapy. She does allow herself to be followed by myself on an occasional basis."

4. Physician's response when asked for any impression of why the patient did better than anticipated:

"She was unusual in that she was very anti-M.D. and establishment, and could not accept the need of radiation. She quit just as she was showing improvement, I suspect on a family member's advice, and started 'diet therapy.' She has exceeded my expectation of survival considering inadequate treatment but remains well. Her struggle was against her M.D.s, including myself, and against her cancer which lead to an unusual combination of unorthodox treatment and conventional treatment. She continues to struggle in an unresolved situation."

[**Author's Comment:** This questionnaire was completed approximately five years ago. Her situation is no longer considered unresolved.]

BETTY PRESTON

1. Estimating the probability of the patient's course of illness:

The physician indicated that the likelihood of her course of illness was approximately 1 in 100. [**Author's note:** Since the most unusual aspect of her illness has been the extent of her recovery from significant brain damage, the physician was asked to estimate the probability of her course of illness rather than the probability of survival.]

2. The physician's description of the patient's illness and treatment:

"1975——Severe brain damage during open heart surgery
Complication: Loss of half of vision
                    Expressive/receptive aphasia"

[In a telephone conversation, this cardiologist also reported: "The heart lung machine was hooked up inappropriately; rather than pulling blood out of one part and putting it into another, they actually pumped air into her blood vessels so the air went up into her head. She wound up with very severe brain damage. . . . She was having seizures for a week or ten days. I told her family that she would have serious brain damage."]

3. Physician's response when asked for any impression of why the patient did better than anticipated:

"Highly motivated
Strong religious beliefs
Strong positive outlook
Strong family support"

[In the phone conversation, the physician also said: "She was always highly motivated. Even at her most desperate times she always had a smile on her face and a positive outlook. She was going to make the most of whatever the situation was."]

REFERENCES

W. Allen. *Side Effects*. New York: Ballantine, 1975.

American Cancer Society. *Cancer Facts & Figures—1988*. New York, 1988.

American Psychiatric Association. *Quick Reference to the Diagnostic Criteria from Diagnostic and Statistical Manual of Mental Disorders*, 3rd ed. Washington, D.C., 1980.

A. A. Amkraut and G. F. Solomon. "Stress and Murine Sarcoma Virus- (Moloney-) Induced Tumors." *Cancer Research*, July 1972, *32*, 1428–33.

C. D. Aring. "Intimations of Mortality." *Annals of Internal Medicine*, July 1968, *69*, 137–152.

Usharbudh Arya. *Meditation and the Art of Dying*. Honesdale, PA: Himalayan Publications, 1975.

D. Ayman. "An Evaluation of Therapeutic Results in Essential Hypertension." *Journal of the American Medical Association*, 1930, *95*, 246–249.

R. W. Bartrop, L. Lazarus, E. Luckhurst, L. G. Kiloh, and R. Penny. "Depressed Lymphocyte Function after Bereavement." *Lancet*, 1977, *1*, 834–836.

E. Becker. *The Denial of Death*. New York: The Free Press, 1973.

M. S. Belsky and H. Gross. *How to Choose and Use Your Doctor.* Greenwich, Conn.: Fawcett, 1975.

H. H. Benjamin. *From Victim to Victor.* Los Angeles: Jeremy P. Tarcher, 1987.

H. Benson and M. Z. Klipper. *The Relaxation Response.* New York: Avon, 1976.

R. A. Berté. *To Speak Again: Victory Over Cancer.* Agawam, Mass.: Phillips Publishing, 1987.

B. G. Braun. "Psychophysiologic Phenomena in Multiple Personality and Hypnosis." *American Journal of Clinical Hypnosis,* October 1983, 124–137.

M. Buber. *Tales of the Hasidim: Later Masters.* New York: Schocken, 1948.

R. J. Bulman and C. B. Wortman. "Attributions of Blame and Coping in the 'Real World': Severe Accident Victims React to Their Lot." *Journal of Personality and Social Psychology,* 1977, *35,* 351–363.

B. R. Cassileth, E. J. Lusk, D. S. Miller, L. L. Brown, and C. Miller. "Psychosocial Correlates of Survival in Advanced Malignant Disease." *New England Journal of Medicine,* 1985, *312,* 1551–55.

N. Cousins. *Anatomy of an Illness.* New York: W. W. Norton, 1979.

N. Cousins. *The Healing Heart.* New York: W. W. Norton, 1983.

N. Cousins. *Human Options.* New York: W. W. Norton, 1981.

C. Delbo. *None of Us Will Return,* trans. by John Githens. New York: Grove Press, 1968.

T. Des Pres. *The Survivor: An Anatomy of Life in the Death Camps.* New York: Oxford University Press, 1976.

R. A. DiOrio. *The Man Beneath the Gift.* New York: Quill, 1981.

R. W. Dubois and R. H. Brook. "Preventable Deaths: Who, How Often, and Why?" *Annals of Internal Medicine,* October 1, 1988, 582–589.

L. Feinberg. "Fire-walking in Ceylon." *The Atlantic Monthly,* May 1959, *203,* 73–76.

T. Ferguson (ed.). *Medical Self-Care.* New York: Summit Books, 1980.

J. Fielding et al. "An Interim Report of a Prospective Randomized, Controlled Study of Adjuvant Chemotherapy in Operable Gastric Cancer: British Stomach Cancer Group." *World Journal of Surgery,* 1983, *7,* 390–399.

J. D. Frank. *Persuasion and Healing.* Baltimore: Johns Hopkins University Press, 1974.

M. Frankenhauser et al. "Psychological Reactions to Two Different Placebo Treatments." *Scandinavian Journal of Psychology*, 1963, *4*, 245–250.

G. Gallup, Jr. *Adventures in Immortality*. New York: McGraw-Hill, 1982.

J. Glassman. "Beating the Odds." *New Age Journal*, November 1985.

J. Glassman. *The Cancer Survivors: And How They Did It*. New York: Doubleday, 1983.

M. L. Gold. "The Relationship of Psychosocial Factors to Prognostic Indicators in Cutaneous Malignant Melanoma." *Journal of Psychosomatic Research*, 1985, *29* (2), 139–153.

J. Goodwin, W. C. Hunt, C. R. Key, and J. M. Samet. "The Effect of Marital Status on Stage, Treatment, and Survival of Cancer Patients." *Journal of the American Medical Association*, December 4, 1987, *258* (21), 3215–30.

S. Greer, T. Morris, and K. W. Pettingale. "Psychological Response to Breast Cancer: Effect on Outcome." *Lancet*, 1979, *11*, 785–787.

S. Hoffman, K. E. Paschkis, and A. Cantarow. "Exercise, Fatigue and Cancer Growth." *Federation Proceedings*, March 1960, *19* (abstracts), 396.

"Hospital Study Cites Preventable Deaths." *The New York Times*, October 2, 1988, 31.

Y. Ikemi, S. Nakagawa, T. Nakagawa, and S. Mineyasu. "Psychosomatic Consideration on Cancer Patients Who Have Made a Narrow Escape from Death." *Dynamic Psychiatry*, 1975, *75*, 77–92.

Institute of Noetic Sciences. "Placebo: The Hidden Asset in Healing." *Investigations*, 1985, *2*, 1–32.

J. Ireland. *Life Wish*. Boston: Little, Brown, 1987.

B. J. Kennedy, A. Tellegen, S. Kennedy, and N. Havernick. "Psychological Response of Patients Cured of Advanced Cancer." *Cancer 38*, 2184–91.

J. Kiecolt-Glaser et al. "Psychosocial Modifiers of Immunocompetence in Medical Students." *Psychosomatic Medicine*, 1984, *46* (1), 7–14.

D. M. Kissen. "The Significance of Personality in Lung Cancer in Men." *Annals of the New York Academy of Sciences*, 1966, *125*, 820–826.

S. B. Kopp. *If You Meet the Buddha on the Road, Kill Him!* New York: Bantam, 1985.

E. Kübler-Ross. "Foreword," in K. Ring, *Heading Toward Omega: In Search of the Meaning of the Near-Death Experience*. New York: William Morrow, 1984.

R. Lamerton. "How Hospices Cope," in D. Horan and D. Mall (eds.), *Death, Dying and Euthanasia*. Washington, D.C.: University Publications of America, 1977.

Lao Tsu. *Tao Te Ching*, trans. by Gia-Fu Feng and Jane English. New York: Vintage, 1972.

R. J. Leider. *The Power of Purpose*. New York: Ballantine, 1985.

L. Le Shan. *The Mechanic and the Gardener*. New York: Holt, Rinehart and Winston, 1982.

L. LeShan. *You Can Fight for Your Life*. New York: M. Evans, 1980.

L. LeShan and M. Reznikoff. "A Psychological Factor Apparently Associated with Neoplastic Disease." *Journal of Abnormal and Social Psychology*, 1960, *60*, 439–440.

L. LeShan and R. Worthington. "Some Recurrent Life History Patterns Observed in Patients with Malignant Diseases." *Journal of Nervous Mental Disorders*, 1956, *124*, 460–465.

S. Levine. *Healing into Life and Death*. Garden City, N.Y.: Anchor Press/Doubleday, 1987.

S. M. Levy, J. Lee, C. Bagley, and M. Lippman. "Survival Hazards Analysis in Recurrent Breast Cancer Patients: Seven Year Follow-up." *Psychosomatic Medicine* L (5), Sept./Oct. 1988.

S. Locke and D. Colligan. *The Healer Within: The New Medicine of Mind and Body*. New York. E. P. Dutton, 1986.

N. L Mages and G. A. Mendelshon. "Effects of Cancer on Patients' Lives: A Personological Approach." In G. Stone, F. Cohen, N. E. Adler, and Associates (eds.), *Health Psychology: A Handbook*. Washington, D.C.: Jossey-Bass, 1979, pp. 255–284.

R. May. *Love and Will*. New York: W. W. Norton, 1969.

K. Menninger. *The Vital Balance*. New York: Viking, 1963.

S. Milgram. "Some Conditions of Obedience and Disobedience to Authority." *Humar Relations*, 1965, *18* (1), 57–76.

R. Moody, Jr. *Life After Life*. Atlanta: Mockingbird Books, 1975.

M. R. Otis. "Psychological Predictors of Recovery from Thoracotomy in Patients with Lung Cancer." *Dissertation Abstracts International*, 1980, *40*, 3959B.

J. C. Pearce. *The Crack in the Cosmic Egg*. New York: Julian Press, 1971, 1988.

K. R. Pelletier. *Mind as Healer, Mind as Slayer: A Holistic Approach to Preventing Stress Disorder*. New York: Delacorte, 1977.

K. R. Pelletier. *Toward a Science of Consciousness*. New York: Delacorte, 1978.

G. Porter and P. A. Norris. *Why Me?* Walpole, N.H.: Stillpoint Publishing, 1985.

Ram Dass. *Journey of Awakening: A Meditator's Guidebook.* New York: Bantam, 1978.

Ram Dass and P. Gorman. *How Can I Help?* New York: Knopf, 1987.

C. P. Richter. "On the Phenomenon of Sudden Death in Animals and Man." *Psychosomatic Medicine,* 1957, *19,* 191–198.

K. Ring. *Heading Toward Omega: In Search of the Meaning of the Near-Death Experience.* New York: William Morrow, 1984.

M. Sabom. *Recollections of Death.* New York: Harper & Row, 1982.

S. J. Schleifer, S. E. Keller, M. Camerino, J. C. Thornton, and M. Stein. "Suppression of Lymphocyte Stimulation Following Bereavement." *Journal of the American Medical Association,* 1983, *250,* 374–377.

A. H. Schmale, Jr., and H. P. Iker. "The Affect of Hopelessness and the Development of Cancer: I? Identification of Uterine Cervical Cancer in Women with Atypical Cytology." *Psychosomatic Medicine,* 1966, *28,* 714–721.

R. Selzer. *Mortal Lessons.* New York: Simon and Schuster, 1974.

R. B. Shekelle et al. "Psychological Depression and 17-Year Risk of Death from Cancer." *Psychosomatic Medicine,* 1981, *43* (2), 117–125.

B. S. Siegel. *Love, Medicine & Miracles.* New York: Harper & Row, 1986.

I. Silvertsen and A. W. Dahlstrom. "Relation of Muscular Activity to Carcinoma: Preliminary Report." *Journal of Cancer Research,* 1921, *6,* 365–378.

O. C. Simonton, S. Matthews-Simonton, and J. L. Creighton. *Getting Well Again.* Los Angeles: J. P. Tarcher, 1978.

L. S. Sklar and H. Amisman. "Stress and Coping Factors Influence Tumor Growth." *Science,* August 1979, *205,* 513–515.

D. W. Smith. "Survivors of Serious Illness." *American Journal of Nursing,* March 1979, 441–446.

Gary Smith. "Just Pray for Me, Baby." *Sports Illustrated,* June 20, 1988, 65–70.

S. Suzuki. *Zen Mind, Beginner's Mind.* New York: Weatherhill, 1970.

L. Temoshok, B. W. Heller, R. Sagebiel, M. Blois, D. Sweet, R. J. DiClemente, M. Gold. "The Relationship of Psychosocial Factors to Prognostic Indicators in Cutaneous Malignant Melanoma." *Journal of Psychosomatic Research,* 1985, *29* (2), 139–153.

C. B. Thomas, and K. R. Duszynski. "Closeness to Parents and the Family Constellation in a Prospective Study of Five Disease States: Suicide, Mental Illness, Malignant

Tumor, Hypertension, and Coronary Heart Disease." *The Johns Hopkins Medical Journal,* 1974, *134,* 251–270.

C. B. Thomas. "Precursors of Premature Disease and Death: The Predictive Potential of Habits and Family Attitudes." *Annals of Internal Medicine.* 87, 1976.

C. B. Thomas, K. R. Duszynski, and J. W. Shaffer. "Family Attitudes Reported in Youth as Potential Predictors of Cancer." *Psychosomatic Medicine,* 1979, *41,* 287–302.

D. C. van Baalen and M. J. de Vries. "Spontaneous Regression of Cancer." Erasmus University, Rotterdam, Netherlands, 1987.

R. von Oech. *A Whack on the Side of the Head.* New York: Warner, 1983.

C. Weinstock. "Recent Progress in Cancer Psychobiology and Psychiatry." *Journal of the American Society of Psychosomatic Dentistry and Medicine,* 1977, *24* (1), 4–14.

T. K. Wilber. "Attitudes and Cancer: What Kind of Help Really Helps?" *Journal of Transpersonal Psychology,* 1988, *20* (1), 49–59.

C. M. Winslow, J. B. Kosecoff, M. Chassin, D. E. Kanouse, and R. H. Brook. "The Appropriateness of Performing Coronary Artery Bypass Surgery." *Journal of the American Medical Association,* July 22/29, 1988, *260* (4), 505–509.

C. B. Wortman and C. Dunkel-Schetter. "Interpersonal Relationships and Cancer." *Journal of Social Issues,* 1979, *35,* 120–155.

INDEX

283